Best Impotence Health Diet: Erectile Dysfunction Health and Diet for Soft Erections

"What you need to do to become a great man again"

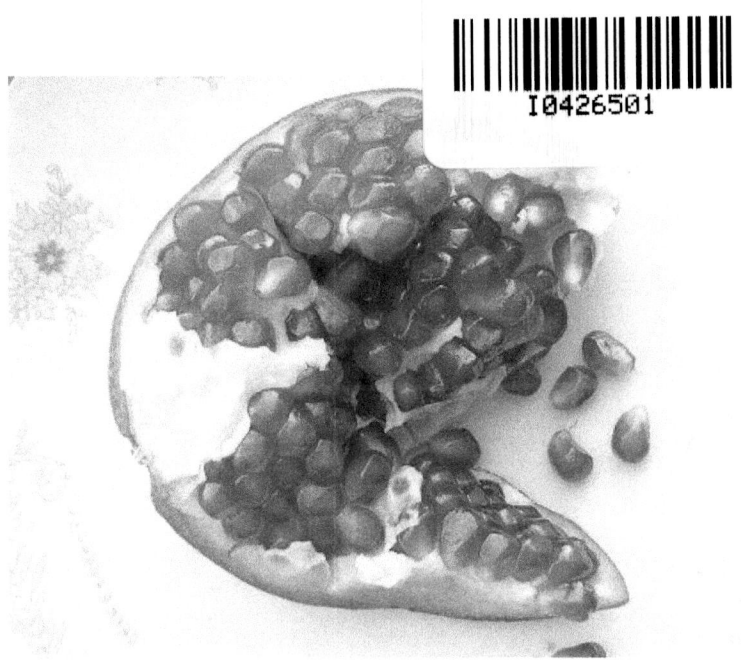

"If you have erectile dysfunction, then you need to examine your lifestyle and make some changes. There is nothing to be ashamed of when you have this condition. There is only one thing for you to do and that is to take action now to correct this condition."

Best Impotence Health Diet: Erectile Dysfunction Health and Diet for Soft Erections © 2012, updated 2018 by Rudy S Silva

Disclaimer and Terms of Use: The Author and Publisher have strived to be as accurate and complete as possible in the creation of this book, notwithstanding the fact that he does not warrant or represent at any time that the contents within are accurate due to the rapidly changing nature of the Internet. While all attempts have been made to verify information provided in this publication, the Author and Publisher assume no responsibility for errors, omissions, or contrary interpretation of the subject matter herein. Any perceived slights of specific persons, peoples, or organizations are unintentional. In practical advice books, like anything else in life, there are no guarantees of income made.

Table of Contents

Table of Contents 5

1: Your Manhood Is On The Line 7

2: Conditions that affect erections or hardness 17

3: Where To Start For Harder Erections 25

4: Diet For Improving Manhood And Losing Weight 37

5: Nutrients That Change You Into A Real Man 49

6: Fruits To Drink For An Alkaline Body 59

7: The Best Fruits That Make You Alkaline 73

8: The Best Vegetables That Make You Alkaline 85

9: Why You Should Drink Vegetable Juices 91

10: Foods That Take Your Manhood Away 113

11: Nutrients That Change You Into A Real Man... 119

12: The Heart Of A Real Man, The Key To Hardness 141

13: Exercises That Increase Your Male Performance 151

14: Natural Body Cycles That Help You Become A Man 158

15: How To Cleanse Your Colon For Sexual Health 175

16: A System To Eliminate Erectile Dysfunction 185

17: The Author And Other Great Resources 193

1: Your Manhood Is On The Line

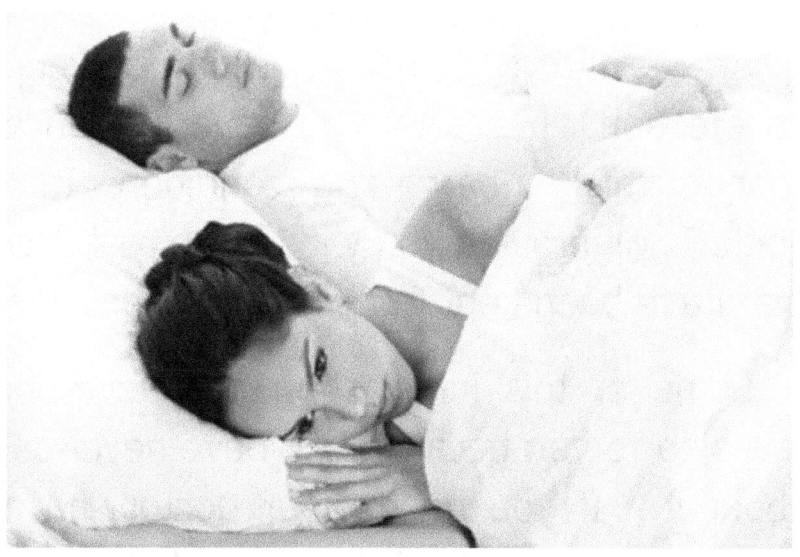

It is said that 10% of males cannot get an erection. Sales for Viagra have skyrocketed to over 2 billion dollars. Males are still using Viagra and other stimulators even though there are dangerous side effects with some deaths reported.

In the past, impotence was blamed mostly on psychological problems, fear of failure, or feelings of inadequacy. But new light has shown that impotence is more related to diet or the illnesses related to poor diet and lifestyle. Sure, psychological issues are sometimes a factor, but diet and lifestyle take the lead.

Are having a hard time getting or keeping an erection? So now, you have a chance to change this embarrassing condition. In this book, I will provide you with some real secrets that have been kept from you for a long time.

Some of this information has never been revealed to you because you have never asked about it. If you go to your doctor, he may give you some of this information but not all of it.

Your doctor, most likely, will recommend the use of drugs as Viagra, Cialis, or Levitra. These drugs have side effects. If you have seen your doctor and are working with him to regain your manhood, then the information here will be of great value.

Viagra works to increase your blood level of nitric oxide and to relax the muscle in your penis so that blood can flow into your penis to make it hard.

The side effects of these drugs are small visual changes, headache, some stomach issues, and flushing.

If you have hardness problems, you may not have erectile dysfunction or impotence. By knowing what to change in your lifestyle, you can regain your hardness and perform like you have in the past.

Your Manhood

But, now that your manhood is on the line, you need to know and do something to get it back. You have, on your computer screen or on your e-reader, information that will transform you into a natural man; a man that you were, when you were in your twenties. Could this get you excited?

Don't fall for those doctors' recommendation of Penile Injection Therapy where you get drugs injected directly into your penis. This is not the way to correct your issue. Or, have you heard of a penis implant, where an inflatable balloon device and a pump are surgically implanted. When you want an erection, you simply pump air into the balloon. Does this sound like a solution to your hardness problem?

In this book, I want you to have a good understanding as to why you may have an erection problem. Of course, these are the things that a doctor should be discussing with you. But, then he would write you a prescription for a nervous condition or for your heart. But, in the end, he should also be telling you to seek out a good nutritionist or alternative practitioner to get solid information on a good manhood diet and health program.

But, at first, the doctor may want to put you on special medication; the drugs that he farms out to all of his patients. But, you may want to avoid these potent chemicals, especially Viagra, that will only make your erection condition worse, over the long run.

And, you know that drugs have side effects, so they may end up killing you slowly. Sometimes the side effects are the very thing you are trying to change or correct.

There is no doubt that if you want to be a man again, you need to get your penis hard and keep it hard while you perform your sexual obligation. This is what you will discover in this book.

How You Got Where You Are Now

There will be a time when you start to see a change in the hardness you get. This can come slowly or suddenly. These changes can be both related to a mental or psychological condition. And, it can be coupled with a physical change in your body. It can also be related to a particular disease that you have or drug that you're using.

As you age, you are susceptible to a variety of diseases that with proper early lifestyle changes could have been prevented. These health issues that you will face later in life or are facing now are cardiovascular disease, stroke, or diabetes. It is these diseases that have the most effect on what type of erections you have or will have – hard or soft.

Weaknesses in your heart muscles and plaque buildup in your artery walls are reflected in the level of penis hardness you can achieve.

How To Get Hard

If you wish to increase and improve your hardness, then you need to improve your health, especially your cardiovascular health. So when your veins, blood, and heart are healthy, so will your brain and body. This results in strong erections.

When your brain creates excitement and causes a release of loads of nitric oxide from the walls of your arteries, your erections will be hard and strong. In addition, if your testosterone levels are normal and your weight is typical, you can expect to get hard easier. Being overweight takes a toll on your heart and your overall cardiovascular health.

The thing to understand here is that good health and a strong erection go hand in hand. Smoking, drinking, diseases such as diabetes, heart issues, emotional troubles and many others diseases or conditions, all have an effect on the level of hardness you can achieve.

Restore Your Hardness

So, if you noticed that you are losing your hardness, it is critical that you start immediately to regain your ability to get hard. Waiting for a long period before you do, can result in procedures that are not as attractive – drugs or surgery.

The purpose of this book is to help you get into sexual shape to restore your lost hardness. Also, it is to get you back into good physical shape and into a healthy condition, so that you can maintain hardness during your sexual activities. The purpose is also to help you keep your hardness and endurance during your sexual activity until you and your partner are satisfied.

Getting your hardness back is the same thing as getting back your health. This will require you to learn and discover the many ways that you can regain your health. It may require you to accept some natural cures and remedies that can balance who you are.

The list below gives you an idea of what can affect your ability to reach different levels of hardness:

- Age
- Health level
- Diet
- Exercise
- Stress
- Mental state, confidence
- Drugs

- Illnesses

- Depression

- Fatigue

- Alcohol

- Marital problems

- Smoking

- Lack of testosterone

- Pituitary tumors

- Hormonal imbalances

Impotence is associated with getting old only because you might have a decline in your health. If you maintain a good lifestyle, which includes a decent diet and exercise, then you should have a minimum of issues with impotence.

2: Conditions that affect erections or hardness

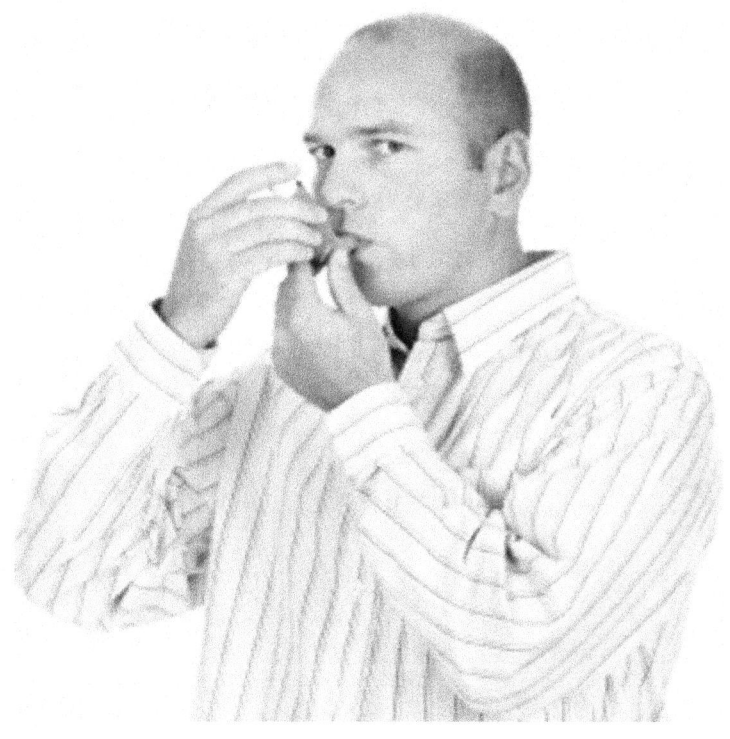

Let's go into more detail as to why you can have problems with erections. There are really a lot of reasons for not getting hard. What your reason is just you know and only your body can correct.

As you age your ability to create an erection diminishes. Now, this not true for all men, in general, but with each passing decades, you can expect your hardness to lessen. Now, what is the cause of this change in your manhood?

The list below is what affects your ability to reach a different level of hardness:

- Age and Activity
- Medications you are using
- Cardiovascular and Heart Health
- Exercise level
- Stress in your home or work
- Mental state or the type of personality you have
- Diseases you may be fighting or that are starting to show up
- The level of health you have had in the past and now
- How you rest and what kind of sleep you get

- Diet habits – the foods you ate in the past and eat now
- Prostate surgery or prostate enlargement
- Cirrhosis of the liver – reduces testosterone in the blood
- Decrease in testosterone

Your erections are not only affected by the list above, but by numerous factors that affect every aspect of your life.

There is no magic pill to improve your sex life. Sure, there is Viagra, Cialis, and Levitra, but these are all classified as drugs. And, you also have a variety of herbal male enhancement products that will help with erections, but using these over the long term is not healthy. For the short term, these can be helpful, since they are not addictive, have few side effects, and can be effective.

When you are young, erections was typically not an issue. You had a strong mind-body connection. You were easily aroused around women, and thinking you would not be able to perform, when in bed with a woman, never entered your mind. It was a given that you would have an erection automatically when the right moment presents itself.

Age and Activity

But, as you age, your confidence about getting hard changes, and soon you begin to feel like you might not be able to get and stay hard.

Your ability to have an erection is critical to who you are. Your hardness is the essence of your manhood. You identify with your erections and your ability to control your hardness and to be able to perform for a woman and to give her and pleasure.

One of the main factors that affect hardness is your age and level of activity. With age comes the emergence of disease. If as you age, you develop heart disease, arteriosclerosis, diabetes, high blood pressure and other major sicknesses, then these conditions affect your ability to have erections.

In some studies in England, it was found that men that had sexual activity three times a week had 50% less cardiovascular problems. The message here is if you are healthy, you can enjoy sex more frequently.

Here is a medical fact: The level of hardness in your erections corresponds to the level of your overall health.

The healthier you are that harder you can get. The softer your erections are the more issues you have with your health.

Medication

The use of drugs has a strong effect on your level of hardness. And, as you continue to use these drugs, the level of point where you have difficulty in creating any hardness.

hardness continues to decrease. Eventually, you can get to the

Drugs that are used to treat hypertension, such as diuretics, tranquilizers or drugs to treat depression also affect hardness.

If you are taking drugs after bypass surgery or other types of surgery, then this will affect your ability to get hard. Many drugs that are used to increase blood circulation or change blood pressure tend to affect hardness.

The use of alcohol and recreational drugs also has a big effect on hardness. This is one area where young men suffer when they entertain themselves with cocaine, heroin, and marijuana. The use of recreational drugs only creates a temporary loss in hardness. Coming off these drugs will return hardness back to normal.

Heart health

In case you don't know it, the condition of your cardiovascular system is directly related to your penis hardness. This is now well documented through research and clinical studies. The pressure from your heart provides the blood and pressure for your erections.

Here's what happens. As you age, plaque starts to build up along your arteries and blood vessel walls. The rate at which this happens depends on your lifestyle. As time passes, the walls start to thicken, because of the plaque buildup.

The first place that this effect is noticed is in your penis hardness. The tiny blood vessels that fill with blood, to make your penis hard, start to become clogged. The walls of these tiny vessels become narrow. And if nothing is done to reverse this condition, you eventually develop erectile dysfunction, a complete lack of ability to produce an erection.

Now, this is why when the signs of lack of hardness start to appear, it is critical that you seek the help of a doctor, who is well versed in helping men who have reduced hardness, have lack of staying power, or that have erectile dysfunction.

The lack of hardness in your penis can be a lifesaver. It is a signal that you have some heart issues that you need to take care before they get too advanced. And since heart issues are not the only factor in this dysfunction, it can be a calling card for other physical or mental issues you need to face and take care.

In this book, you will find a nutritional and lifestyle program that will help you restore the tiny vessels in your penis back to health, so that you can once again feel like a young man.

3: Where To Start For Harder Erections

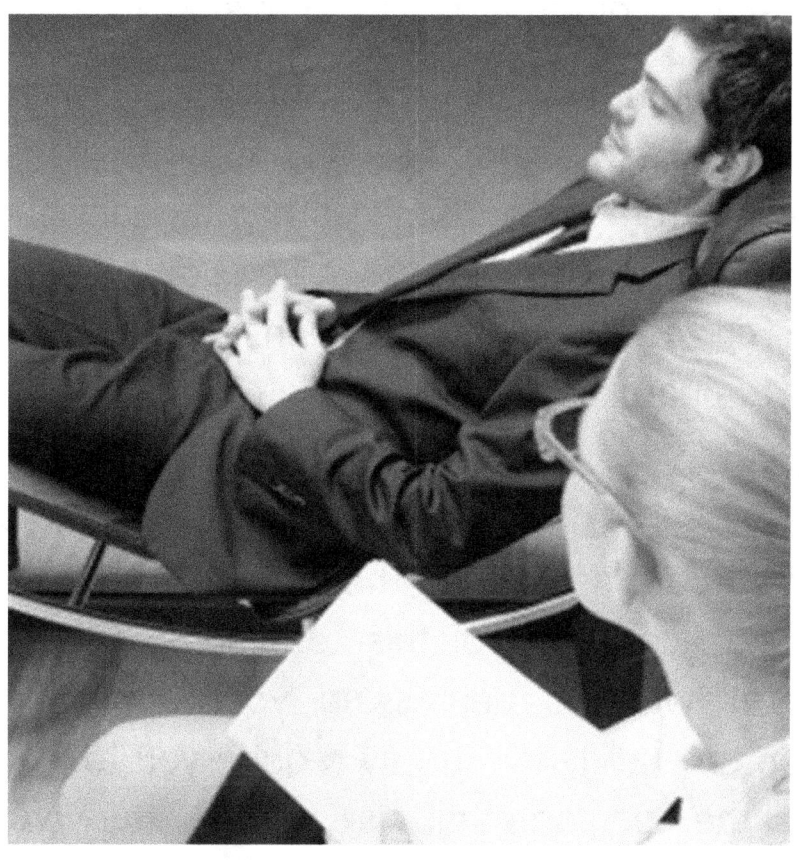

Since having good sex depends on your overall health, you need to be concerned about how to get your health back into better shape. The first place to start with, to improve your hardness, is to look at habits that have a big impact on your sex life. Then make an effort to reduce or eliminate these habits. There are certain reasons why these habits have a big impact, and these will be discussed at different places in this book.

Just keep in mind that not getting hard might be a temporary condition. If it is resulting from stress, such as marital conflicts or work relations with coworkers or bosses, then correcting these situations can relieve your temporary hardness problem.

Stress and Depression

If you are depressed, then you need to find a way to come out of this condition. Take a look at what is depressing you, and take action to change it. It may require you to talk with the person that is related to your depression so that some resolution can occur. Is it some life situation where you feel trapped and can't seem to do anything about it?

If your depression is related to a loved one's death, then you may need to talk to a therapist to help you over this difficult time.

The idea here is when you are stress or depressed you need to take action to solve the problem and not be disabled. Many times it is hard to take this first action, but remember this is affecting your health and hardness, and this is what you want to correct or change.

Smoking, Drugs, and Alcohol

Smoking is probably one of the most devastating habits to have and one of the more difficult ones to stop. When smoking, you are using up a high level of your antioxidants that you need to help you maintain good health in all parts of your body.

When you smoke, you have more plaque buildup in your arteries and veins that limit the amount of blood that flows into your penis to make it hard.

Cirrhosis of the liver from chronic alcoholism can lower the amount of testosterone you have moving through your bloodstream. Testosterone stimulates the sex drive and assists in producing sperm.

Drinking a small amount of wine can be relaxing and contains a high level of anti-oxidants, which are good for your arteries. Studies have shown that only a small amount should be taken every day and that it should not be overdone.

Nitric Oxide

Nitric oxide is a polluting gas outside of your body, but inside your body, nitric oxide, which is produced in the artery walls, is a signaling chemical. When it is released, it gives instructions that control many body functions, such as nerve signals, immune functions, muscle growth and relaxation, blood vessel dilation, and inflammation control.

You will not be able to have erections without producing the proper levels of nitric oxide. Having a good supply of blood to your penis is not enough to have a hard erection. To have a strong erection, you need a good supply of nitric oxide. But that has to be coupled with a good supply of blood to the penis.

To get an erection you need to be stimulated by images, women, or thoughts. These sensations are transmitted to your nervous system, which then triggers the release of nitric oxide. This then relaxes penis muscle, which allows blood to flow into the corpus cavernosum of the penis.

cavernosum. The penis has two shafts called corpus cavernosum as shown in the penis cross section below. It is Nitric Oxide is a gas that is created in the veins of the penis wall, which assists in passing blood into the corpus these shafts that fill with blood when the nervous system relaxes the muscles surrounding the corpora cavernosa.

It is the nitric oxide in the blood that activates the muscles around the corpus cavernosa to relax so that the constricted blood vessels that flow blood into cavernosa can relax and open up.

Without nitric oxide going into the cavernosum no erection is possible.

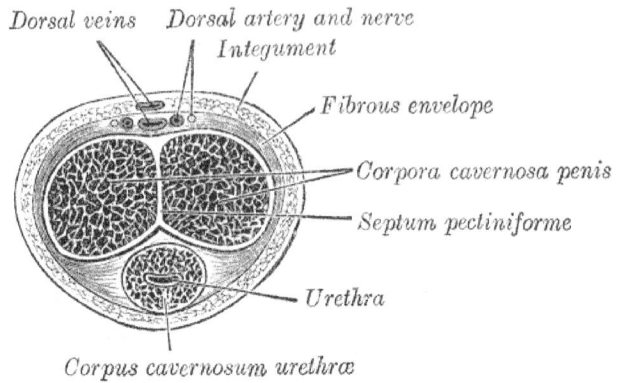

Diagram from Grays' Anatomy

The healthier you are the more Nitric oxide you will produce. This is why you need to concentrate on becoming healthier in all aspects of your life – the foods you eat, the supplements you take, the thoughts you have, and the exercise you do. You need to keep the levels of nitric oxide up throughout your body all the time. This gives you protection against impotency, heart attacks, and other diseases.

Nitric oxide not only functions in your body to give you a hard erection, but it is an important chemical massager that works throughout your body. It works in the cardiovascular system and the central nervous system; it fights infections and works to prevent you from getting ulcers. The list of what nitric oxide does in your body is extremely long.

Many things can interrupt the proper workings of your reproductive system. It can be psychological, physical, or medical. But, it has been found that one of the major causes of erectile dysfunction is the inability to produce enough Nitric Oxide in the corpus cavernosum.

In the following chapters, you will discover how to increase your levels of nitric oxide.

Lifestyle Changes

A relatively healthy body is needed to

create hardness. So the healthier you are the stronger and longer lasting will be your erections. If your health is not so good, this will be reflected in your penis hardness and how long it stays hard.

The level of hardness can vary, so if you get hard but not as hard as you would like, then it's an indication that you need to improve your health. If you get some hardness, but it does not stay hard for very long then again, you need to look at living a healthy lifestyle.

Diet is where you need to start. Being overweight or obese has a direct relationship on how hard you get. You will have to lose some weight if you are overweight. Being overweight is related to a variety of illnesses that can plague you if you maintain that weight or increase that weight.

In the following chapters, you will find suggestions on how to improve your overall health. You will find diets to follow, nutrients that you need, supplement to take, and exercise to do.

All of these suggestions and steps are designed to improve your cardiovascular system, blood circulation, increase nitric oxide, lose weight, and increase mental attitude.

Erectile Dysfunction Psychological or Physical.
If you have this dysfunction, then you might be thinking about whether it is psychological, or if it is due to some physical problem. Here is a test you can use, but it is not full proof.

Every night a man usually gets one or more erections naturally when he sleeps. If you don't get a nightly erection, then your problem might be psychological. If you do get an erection at night, then your problem might be a physical illness.

To determine if you had an erection at night, there is one test used by many. Wrap a strip of postage stamps around the shaft of your penis, before you go to bed. If the strip is in tack in the morning, then you didn't get a nightly erection. You can wrap other things on your penis that can tell if you had an erection.

You may also want to go to your doctor to get a checkup, especially for heart function. If you find that you have heart issues, you can decide whether you want to use drugs or whether you want to use a natural approach for your heart problems and for your erectile dysfunction.

If it is psychological, then you need to discuss this with your partner, so that there no miscommunication between you and her. Most men that are experiencing impotency have lost their confidence in producing erections. It would be a good idea to see a therapist that is versed in this area.

You should also examine areas of your life where you are stressed and have issues with other people that have not been resolved.

One area to start with is your attitude. You need to take control and responsibility for your body. Many men make the mistake of giving their penis a name, like Roger, Biggy, Volcano, Johnny, and so on. The act of giving your penis a name is a process where you are dissociating yourself from your penis. It is like another person to you. It's your penis and you should consider it part of your body and accept that you are having problems with your penis and not that Roger is having problems.

You don't give other parts of your body names, so it does not seem natural to give your penis a name. Changing your attitude in this area will help you start to consider that your whole body has to change, including the way you think about your penis.

4: Diet For Improving Manhood And Losing Weight

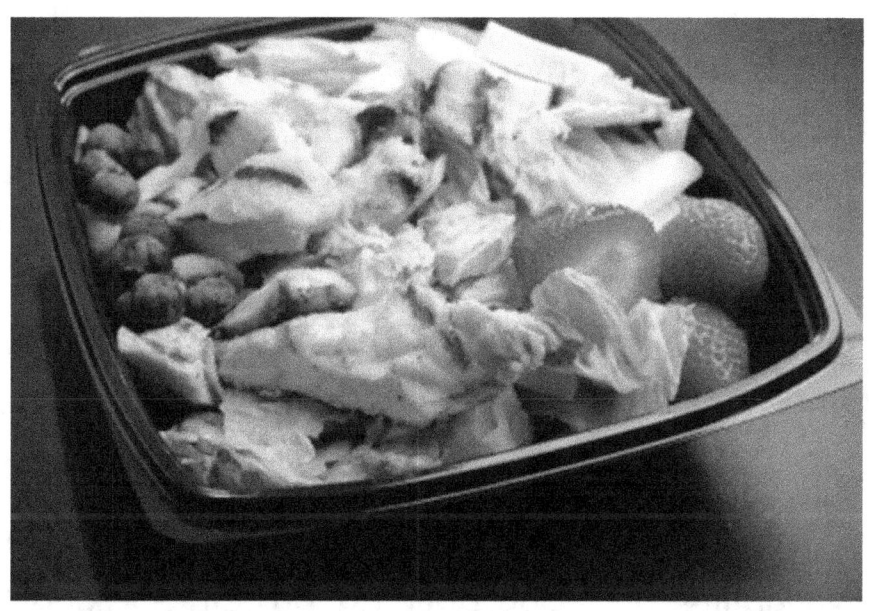

Amino Acids

Eating to get all the amino acids, essential or nonessential, is necessary for maintaining your manhood. Your protein can come from meat, grains, or vegetables. What is important is that you get all the essential amino acids and they don't all have to come from the same meal. You can get them during different meals in one day. Your body will store them and wait for the missing ones to show up. But they have to be in enough quantity so that the amino acids can start their work on building your body.

The lack of any one of the amino acids will thwart the process of amino cell and muscle building.

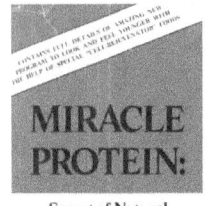

In his book, Carlson Wade, Miracle Protein: Secret of Natural Cell-Tissue Rejuvenation, Park Publishing, 1975, writes,

"Cell therapists claim that the availability of tissue-building protein to repair and replace fragments of the body's building blocks can do more than extend the prime of life. Cellular nutrition and can help create extended sexual potency. The availability of a balanced amount of amino acids can create an environment that will help nourish the cells and tissues of those body components involved with better virility in the male and more healthful sexual desires in the female.

Cell therapists who specialize in nutrition for youthful vigor have suggested that a food program emphasize a balance of all important nutrients and a balance of all protein foods. The amino acids can then work harmoniously to create an extended and prolonged sexual desire for protein-ized males and females."

Foods You Should Be Eating

- Protein
- Fruit juices
- Fruits
- Vegetable juices
- Vegetables
- Grains
- Seed and nuts
- Good Oils
- Water

Protein

Protein has an enormous effect on your ability to maintain and keep your sexual abilities active and strong. Your body converts protein into amino acids that help feed the cells and tissues that are part of your sexual function. Your cells are nourished, repaired, and energized keeping you young and active.

However, eating excess meat is harmful to your health. Eating too much meat, more than 2-4 ounces per day, has been found to contribute to the narrowing of the arteries. And, if you are lacking in certain B vitamins, you open yourself to plaque buildup along your artery walls.

If you do physical labor and are involved in a lot of movement in your work, then you should eat more than 2-4 protein ounces per day. Just make sure that the meat has a minimum of additives and preservatives.

Remember, meat is high in saturated fat, which blocks the activity of essential fatty acids, EPA and DHA, found in fish oil, which controls the activity of your hormones.

Here is where you need to get your protein.

Lean meats and liver - Buy the meat products that are free ranged or organically raised. Such meat has little or no growth hormone injections or un-natural injections.

Seeds and nuts – are high in protein and zinc and have an influence on your prostate gland, which needs to be in good health for good sex performance.

Whole grains - have a lot of protein, minerals, and vitamins that support the formation and secretion of testosterone. One of the prime grains to eat is unprocessed oat. Don't use the quick oats, they are depleted of nutrients. Real oats will provide you with the protein and minerals to get you hard. Eat these every day, with various fruits listed below, every other day or for a few weeks. You want to follow the body cycle listed in Chapter 9.

Meat and Bread

Meat and bread is a big contributor to creating constipation.   Meat is difficult to digest, and many times it will get into the colon partial digested. This condition benefits the bad bacteria and allows them to dominate the colon, which creates constipation.

Because meat and bread have little fiber, they move slowly in the colon, which leads to constipation and eventually to some type of colon inflammation.   For this reason, you should always eat a salad when you eat these foods. Having constipation lessens your desire to have sexual encounters.

Bad bacteria, decaying meat, and other undigested food contribute to the buildup of toxic matter in the colon. You need matter in the colon to move daily out the rectum, otherwise, toxic matter will build up and end up in your bloodstream, creating a variety of sickness.

A toxic colon is not able to function right. It is not able to eliminate toxins out through your stools.   So what happens is the toxic matter gets into your bloodstream, and it comes out in your breath and through the pores of your skin. This is one reason you could have body order.

How Protein Helps Your Sexual Hardness

Protein or amino acids tend to refresh cells and tissues by removing waste products that are created by cell metabolism. When you have a clean body inside and out, you will have a stronger desire to have sex and the ability to perform.

Protein tends to smooth out your metabolism, which allows you to have longer and harder sex. A fast body metabolism burns you out fast, leaving you with unsatisfied sexual encounters.

Glutathione, the master antioxidant, is formed from amino acids. It is this nutrient that extends your life by fighting and neutralizing free radicals inside and outside of your cells. It helps to reduce the plaque buildup along your arteries that can block the release of nitric oxide.

Protein is a cell and tissue rebuilder. Wherever you have broken down, dead, or damaged cells and tissue, these cells need to be replaced or rebuilt. Without your ability to replace damaged cells, your sexual strength will be compromised. Body stress of any kind breaks down cells and tissue. It is critical that these cells be repaired.

Damage to cells also comes from cross-linking. This cross-linking comes from molecules that connect improperly when exposed to the sun, pollution and other unhealthy environments.

One of the most powerful activities of protein is to keep your cells ventilated so that oxygen flows freely, allowing it to create the energy you need for your sexual activities.

Natural Sex Drink

Here is juice drink you can prepare to give you protein and a balance of minerals and vitamins.

- 8 oz. of cherry or pomegranate juice
- 2 tablespoons of brewer's yeast
- 2 tablespoons of wheat germ
- 4 tablespoons of desiccated liver

Stir until mixed properly. Drink three glasses each day – morning, noon and night.

Yeast has all of the amino acids that your body needs.

This drink has a direct effect on cell-tissue regeneration and replication. It has a strong effect in the sexual centers of your body, eventually providing you with additional strength to power up your sexual desire and organ. Try this out for 5 to 7 day and see your life change.

Here are more sources of protein that you need to add to your diet.

Soybeans – if you can eat cooked soybeans with brown rice, this will improve your sexual desire. Soybean powder is also available and can be used to make smoothies.

The liver is a good food for protein. If you like liver, look for a liver that comes from organic farm animals. Or, you can get liver powder and add it to your smoothies.

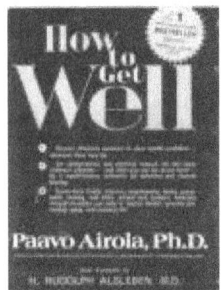

Nuts are high in protein and minerals, which help to nourish the ovaries. Nuts can be eaten as snacks between meals. Use almonds, pine nuts, pecans, walnuts, and cashews, pumpkin seeds. Eat these nuts raw to get the best nutritional value from them. Use them as between meal snacks.

Whole grains provide a lot of protein, and they help in producing testosterone. Fish contains protein and minerals that help rebuild brain cells.

Paavo Airola, Ph.D., in his book How to Get Well, Health Plus, Publishers, 1974, lists a sex Pep-up Cocktail which makes two glasses,

- "1 ½ glasses of whole, raw, unpasteurized milk
- 2 tbsp., non-instant skim milk powder
- 2 egg yolks, raw or whole eggs can use
- 1 tbsp. wheat germ oil – only if available fresh, non-rancid

Otherwise, use cold-pressed sesame seed oil or olive oil

2 tbs. wheat germ-if available fresh, not more than one week old

- 1 tbsp., sesame seeds
- 2 tbsp., pumpkin seeds
- 2 tsp., lecithin granules
- 1 tbsp., natural, raw honey
- 1 tbsp., crushed ice

Grind the sesame and pumpkins seed in a coffee grinder first. Then blend all ingredients in the blender. Eat slowly with a spoon, or sip through a straw.

This is a perfect lunch for a busy, tired husband. A perfect revitalizing drink for a tired wife, too."

Look over the ingredients in this Pep-up drink and use replacement where necessary. The important thing is to get as many of the ingredients called for.

5: Nutrients That Change You Into A Real Man

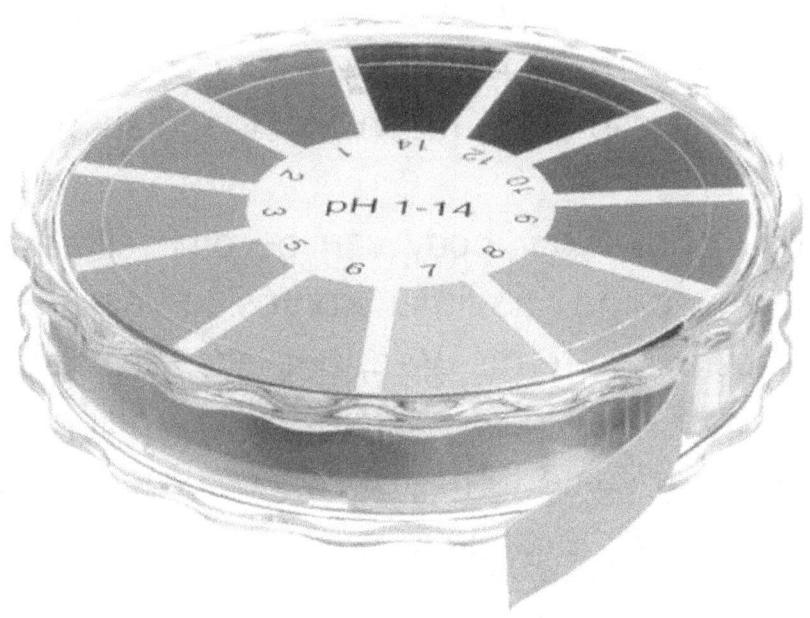

Minerals

Moving your body more toward alkalinity is what will give you the best curative effects of fruits. An alkaline body prevents your body from becoming ill and forming deadly diseases, like all kinds of joint problems, organ degradation, body pain, heart disease, or even cancer. If you are already sick, then all the chemicals inside fruits will help to revive you to better health. This is provided that your tissue damage has not gone beyond repair.

The minerals most importance in changing and maintaining your body in an alkaline condition are sodium,potassium, chloride, calcium, phosphorus, magnesium, and sulfur.

Now, how your body can become alkaline might become a little confusing at first because of the terms used, but let's break this down into small parts. First, we are going to be defining some terms, so we can then start talking the same language.

Acid Binding

There are certain minerals that are called acid binding. And these are minerals we said are the most important ones in fruits, Sodium, potassium, chloride, calcium, phosphorus, magnesium, because they are acid binding.

What acid binding means is when you eat fruits with these minerals, they will seek out acids in your body and combine with them to neutralize them, by creating a new chemical called alkaline forming ash.

Alkaline Ash

After this alkaline forming ash has tied up an acid, it is carried to the kidney where it is expelled as urine.

Different reactions can occur when an acid-binding mineral, like say sodium, encounters an acid. Of course, acids in the body are toxic, so the body has the priority of getting rid of them fast since they can damage tissue and cause pain and disease.

Here is another pathway of the acid-bindin mineral process, when it combines with an acid.

The Acid Binding Mineral Process

When you eat acid binding food, the blood

carries it to the cells where it is oxidized, digested, or metabolized. The result of this digestion is a carbonic acid salt of alkaline minerals, which reacts with body acids and binds with them. In this process, a weak carbonic acid is created. Now, this weak carbonic acid is taken by the blood into your lungs where it is released as carbon dioxide and water.

If not all the acid toxins are captured by acid binding matter, the remaining acids can be neutralized by body stores of alkaline minerals. If you don't have a good store of alkaline minerals, then these acids will remain in your body creating disease. But if you do have a good store of alkaline minerals, these minerals will find acids, capture them, and bind with them. Then these acids are routed out through your urine and out of your body.

So you can see the importance of getting a lot of alkaline minerals into your body. Without them, acids, which do not get bonded to alkaline minerals, would move back into body tissue and continue their body damage.

Alkaline Binding

Now, there are also minerals that become alkaline binding and these minerals are sulfur, chlorine, iodine, phosphorus, bromine, fluorine, copper, and silicon. It is these minerals that when digested by a cell will produce a salt that will bind with alkaline minerals. These minerals will be excreted through your urine. When alkaline minerals are bonded to an acid salt, the alkaline mineral is removed from your body and your body becomes more acidic, the condition you are trying to avoid.

Although you need to eat both foods that are acid binding or alkaline binding, you want to eat more of the acid-binding foods. This will keep your body slightly alkaline.

Keeping Healthy

One of the most important parts of health is keeping the lymph liquid around your cells clean and free of toxins. To do this you need to provide acid binding minerals to occupy the lymph liquid. These minerals remove the acids that accumulate in your lymph liquid and in all parts of your body tissue.

Body Detoxification

The highest priority of the body is to detoxify itself. One of the best way to help your body detoxify is to provide minerals that bind with acids that are in the cells, tissues, organs, and muscles. What these alkaline acid binding minerals do is to pull out the toxins that are dispersed throughout your body.

These acid binding salts have the ability to suck those acids out and bind with them. But, because not all body chemical reactions follow the same directions, there are times that the alkaline acid binding does not take place.

With the help of the liver, which detoxifies the blood, the kidney removes impurities from the blood and the lungs. The lungs will remove the CO_2, which resulted from alkaline acid binding.

Your body is constantly detoxifying itself. However, when it is overloaded with acid toxins from your lifestyle, a complete detoxification of your body may become impossible.

Where do Acid Toxins Come From?

So why is the body overloaded with toxins? Why can't the liver take care of these toxins? Your liver has the function to remove acid wastes from natural food that is created by food digestion and cell metabolism. When your body encounters acid wastes, such as food enhancers, dyes, preservatives, pesticides, and the variety of additives, the liver does not know how to break them down and to make them harmless.

But, your body does not give up so easily, when it knows that the liver was not able to disintegrate food additives. What it does is it instructs calcium to bind with these toxic acids and to take them far away from the bloodstream.

When calcium binds with acids, a calcium deposit can form in your teeth, and your joints as bone spurs, which grow in your feet or shoulders, vertebra, or muscle tissue. These calcium deposits are very painful, and if you have ever experienced them, you know how much.

Now, we have talked about acid toxins in the body that are brought in through food and the environment. But, there is another factor that creates acid in the body and that is emotions that are activated through life stresses, like work pressures, divorce, friendship problems, marital issues, and other similar problems. These emotional problems create acidic molecules that then embed themselves into your tissues just like food acids

Body Organs

All body organs function to rid the body of acid waste or toxins. Lack of alkaline binding food causes deterioration of the function of these organs. Each organ has a specific function in the elimination and neutralization of acid wastes and it does this in conjunction with alkaline acid binding minerals.

In the next chapter is a list of the fruits that have the highest alkaline minerals and the ones that you should be eating. The percentage assigned to these fruits is based on fresh fruits that are organic, and that they are not cooked, canned or mixed with sugar. If they are a cook or otherwise processed in some fashion, this will reduce their effectiveness as an acid binding fruit.

However, they will still be somewhat effective in acid binding.

6: Fruits To Drink For An Alkaline Body

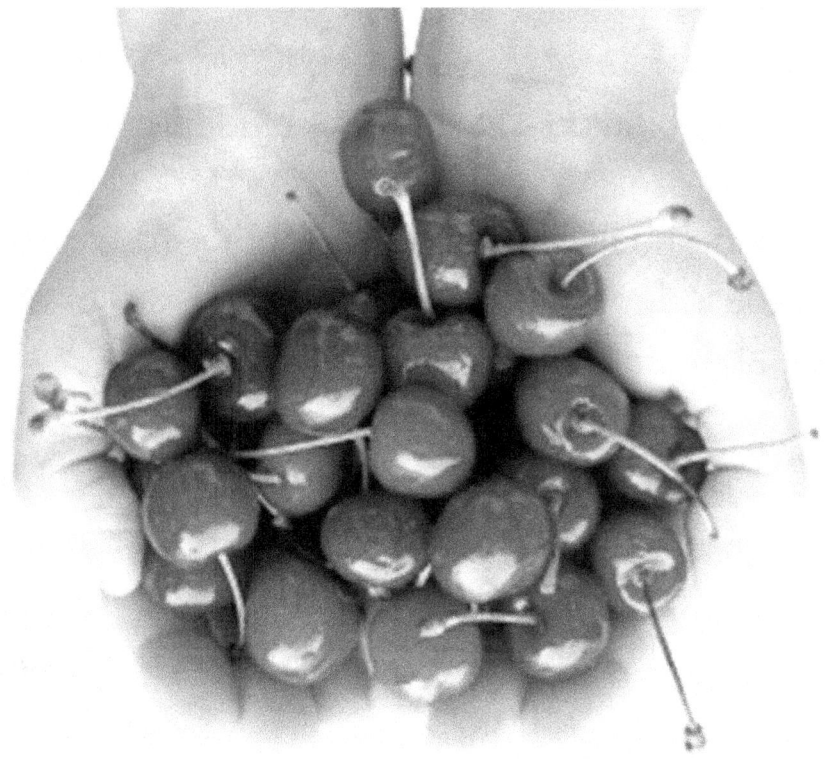

Acid Binding Fruits With Alkaline Minerals

In the list below are fruits with alkaline minerals that create an acid-binding salt your body used to neutralize acid wastes. Fruits above 50% in value are more acid binding, which means they will trap acid wastes better. You will want to eat and drink those fruits above 51%.

The fruits at 50% are neutral. They are not acid binding nor alkaline binding.

You should be eating and drink fruits from all these levels, but eat 80% of the fruits that are above 50%.

Here is the list of fruits to eat and drink in the order of priority.

1. Fruits at 100% Acid Binding – Best fruits To Eat And Drink

Lemons, melons – any type, watermelon

2. Fruits at 93% Acid Binding – Great fruits To Eat And Drink

Cantaloupes, dried dates, dried figs, limes, mango, papaya

3. Fruits at 87% Acid Binding – Still Great Fruits To Eat And Drink

Kiwis, passion fruit, pineapples, raisins, umeboshi plums

4. Fruits at 80% Acid Binding – Eat And Drink These Fruits

Apricots, avocados, bananas, fresh dates, fresh figs, currants, gooseberries grapes, grapefruits guavas, kumquats, nectarines, pears, persimmons, quince

5. Fruits at 73% Acid Binding – Still Fruits To Eat And Drink

Apples, organs, peaches, pomegranate, raspberries, sour grapes, strawberries

6. Fruits at 67% Acid Binding – Still Neutralizes Acids, Eat And Drink This fruit Cherries

Fruits To Concentrate On

These are the fruits you should concentrate on eating. Also, eat them every day, if possible, fresh lemon juice in the morning, watermelon during the day.

You can see which fruits give you the best acid binding effects and eating and drinking them 80% of your overall food intake will convert your body over to an Alkaline body.

Here is another rule. If you eat an acid fruit or acid food like meat which is a 13% and an alkaline binding food that is 80 -100%, you can offset the meat's acids. Don't eat fruit at the same time as your meals. They use different enzymes in your stomach for digestion.

Drinking fruit juices helps to bring vitamins and minerals quickly into your blood. Minerals are the key to keeping your body alkaline. Keeping an alkaline body helps to keep away disease and will strengthen your cardiovascular system.

Juices have antibacterial action and contain digestive enzymes that help you to digest protein and fat. Because of the vitamins, minerals, digestive enzymes, pure water, and nutrients that juices have, they have the power to cleanse your body of toxic wastes, lower your blood pressure, and make your heart stronger.

Try to use organic fruit when making your juice. It is better to make your own juices since most bottled juice contains no life force or natural live enzymes. Drink the juices soon after you juice them. If you want, put them in a thermos for later in the day. If you have no choice but to use store juices, get them bottles instead of plastic. Plastic bottles leach out toxic chemicals.

Here Are Some Juices to Drink.
Apple juice

Drink at least 2 glasses of this juice every day. Apple juice has a high level of minerals and vitamins, which makes it ideal for making your body alkaline.

Apricot – berry juice

Mix equal parts of apricot and berry juice and add a little honey to taste. Drink one cup in the morning. Place the other two glasses into a thermos and drink one more glass at noon and one at dinner.

Berries

Blackberries – help cleanse the blood and are good for constipation. They help a weak kidney and are filled with antioxidants, which fight plaque buildup in your arteries.

Cherry juice

Cherry juice is a powerful drink. Because it has so many minerals, it will make your body more alkaline by neutralizing acid waste in the blood, in the lymph liquid and wherever it goes. It will also help in keeping you regular. Cherries are good blood cleansers and help the liver and kidney.

Grape Juice

I usually add grape juice to other juices like apple to give it a different flavor. When juicing apples, you can add a few handfuls of grapes to create a new mixture. Grapes have a high content of natural sugar and can give you a quick energy lift. They contain a high level of minerals and have B vitamins.

Many times I will drink this juice from bottles since it has a short season and in a bottle, you can drink it any time. Use the darker grape drinks, because of their high anti-oxidant nutrients

Grapes help to regulate and increase your metabolism. A low metabolism will cause you to gain weight and a high metabolism will help you burn food quicker and get you tired sooner. Because of its mineral content, it helps to build your blood and to stimulate your liver to increase its cleansing abilities. The color of fruit juices often tell you what part of the body it is good for. Red grape juice helps build your blood.

Lemon Juice

Lemon juice is one of the best juices you can drink to help detoxify your liver. It contains many minerals, which will eliminate acid waste. Lemon juice will help constipation, liver disorders, reduce mucus accumulation, improve digestion, reduce infections, and help to clear skin disorders.

One way I use lemon juice is to squeeze the juice of one lemon into 8 oz. of water and drink it first thing in the morning. You can also carry unsweetened lemon water in a thermos and drink it during the day.

Melons

Melon juice is almost the perfect food in that it has many vitamins and minerals. It is most helpful for constipation and kidney and skin disorders. Melons and Cantaloupes are high in vitamin A, C and have many other minerals. Do not eat them with other fruits or juices.

Orange and grapefruit

Prepare half and half of orange and grapefruit juice, using a hand juicer. The flavor is extremely tasty. The combination of these two fresh fruits will give you a powerful start in the morning. They will give you a vitamin C boost with plenty of flavonoids and minerals.

These combined fruits will cleanse your intestinal tract, help in blood disorders, liver disorders, lung disorders, and an acid body condition.

Orange and lemon juice

Mix 3 parts of orange juice with one part lemon juice.

Add a little water and honey and put into a thermos. Drink the juice all day long.

Pineapples

Pineapple juice increases male potency, reduces menstrual cycle issues, and strengthens muscles and tissues. It reduces body acidity and excess bile and strengthens the heart.

Pineapple juice is another excellent juice to use frequently. Its high potassium helps to keep your brain nerve transmission active. Its health value comes from the enzyme bromelain that it contains. Bromelain helps keep body fluids balance and neutral; it moves an acid body to neutral and an alkaline one to neutral. It stimulates the pancreas to release its hormones.

And, it has been found useful for coughs and sore throats. For some people, pineapple juice affects the throat making it feel scratchy.

Pineapples contain many vitamins and minerals. They contain Papain, which helps to digest protein. Pineapples are useful when you have excess mucus, digestive problems, intestinal worms, and constipation.

Pomegranate

Pomegranate juice is one of the best juices to get yourself back to health and for helping you regain your manhood. Pomegranate juice controls bile and phlegm, increases hemoglobin and purifies the blood, and improves appetite, and settles upset stomachs. It restores and sharpens memory, and. It is helpful in many diseases since it neutralizes body acids. It will cure nosebleed by placing a couple drops in each is effective in urinary issues, nose. It is excellent for reducing fever.

Drinking half a glass or more twice a day will help you reduce high blood pressure.

Watermelon

Here is another excellent fruit to eat. Watermelon juice can be obtained by simply eating raw watermelon since it is 98% distilled water. Its use helps cleanse the kidney and bladder since it is a diuretic – removes excess fluids from the body. You can chew on the seeds as you eat watermelon to get extra zinc and vitamin E.

Watermelon juice tones your body prevents heat stroke, normalizes high blood pressure, and strengthens your heart and brain. It helps to cure jaundice and spleen enlargement. It improves digestion, cures chronic headaches, controls nausea and vomiting, calms the nerves, and is a mild laxative.

Eating watermelon in the morning to get its

juice will help you remove a nightly accumulated toxin through your urine. This will you restore kidney function.

7: The Best Fruits That Make You Alkaline

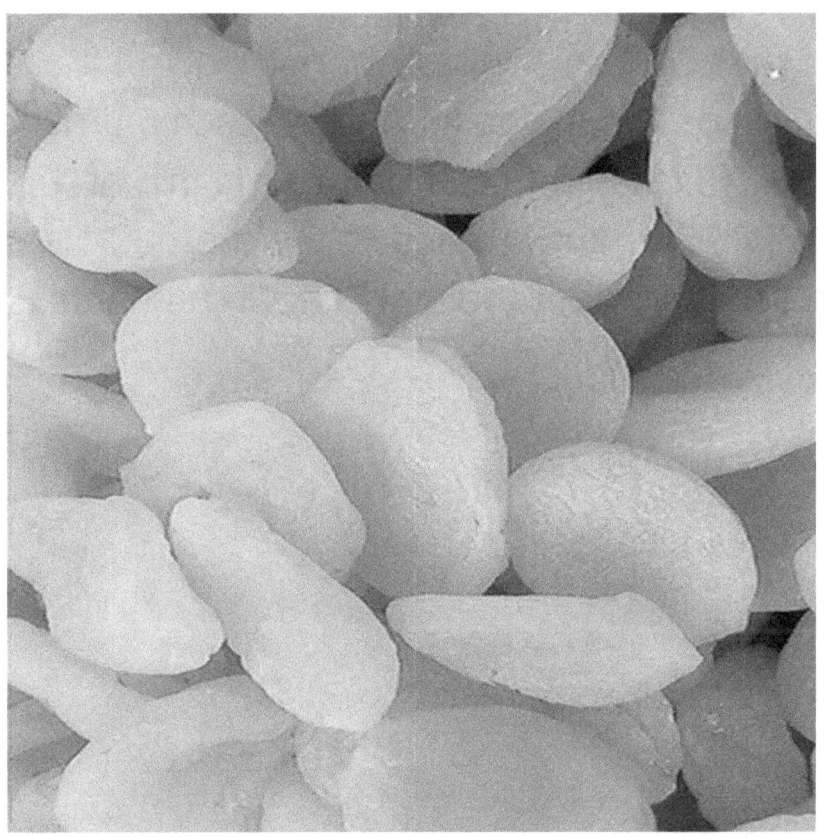

Fruits

Because fruits are naturally grown from the soil, they pull minerals from the ground, and they are a great source of nutrients for you if the soil is heavy with minerals. Because of these minerals and other nutrients, fruits have amazing curative effects, when they are eaten raw. In some cases, it is better to cook them for their healing effects.

Fruits contain a variety of nutrients that are necessary for maintaining life. Each nutrient has a function in your body. Many of the functions are known, and many are not. Here is a list of some of the main known nutrients.

- Minerals
- Antioxidants
- Vitamins
- Fiber
- Natural water
- Enzymes
- Phytonutrients
- Unknown chemicals

Minerals

There are many minerals and vitamins that

are classified as antioxidants. These are vitamins A, C, E, and selenium. Other antioxidants are bioflavonoids, carotenoids, and isoflavones. Vegetables have antioxidants, minerals, and nutrients that cure disease. Your body uses these antioxidants to stop the formation of deadly diseases in your body.

Eat fruits between meals and alternate between drinking them as juice and eating them whole.

Bananas

Eat only one to two banana a day. Bananas have the phytochemicals fructoOligosaccharides, which feeds the good bacteria in your colon. By feeding the good bacteria, you prevent the bad bacteria from overtaking the colon and producing toxic acids.

Bananas are high in potassium and are high in fiber. They are a good source of Folate, vitamin C, and B-6. Bananas contain practically no sodium. However, sodium is one of a top nutrient to consume. But only the sodium in fruits and vegetables is what your body needs.

Apples

Apples are high in soluble fiber, with the skin containing small amounts of beta-carotene. They contain vitamin C, potassium, and some iron. Apples in the morning provide fiber and pectin, which helps to clean out your colon.

You can also eat dried apples, but most nutrients are lost in the drying process except iron and fiber.

Apricots

Apricots have a short season and that is why you see a lot of dried apricots for sale. Eat apricots in season. They are high in beta-carotene, iron, potassium, and vitamin C. They also are high in fiber.

Dried apricots are more nutritious than fresh since the nutrients are more concentrated. The major problem with dried apricots is that they are dried with sulfur dioxide and this creates more acid and health issues in your stomach.

There are some dried apricots that use low sulfur dioxide and some that use no sulfur dioxide.

Avocados

Avocado is a fruit. It is one of the fruits that are highest in mono-unsaturated fatty acid, omega-9, which is a good fat. Most avocado fat consists of 60 - 75% omega-9. It also contains vitamin E, folic acid, fiber and many other nutrients. Omega-9 is an important omega to consume and not many foods contain this nutrient.

Berries

Berries, blackberries, raspberries, and strawberries are high in fiber and antioxidants. The deeper that colors – red, blue, and black - the more antioxidants they have. Antioxidants combine with free radicals in your body to deactivate them.

Free radicals are now considered the molecular ions that cause the most damage to your body. Neutralizing the most free radical in your body is one of your first priorities.

Cantaloupes

Cantaloupe is one of the best fruits to eat. It has a high source of antioxidants, vitamin C, and beta-carotene. It is also high in fiber. Eat cantaloupe only with other melons and do not eat it with other fruits. The stomach enzymes necessary to digest cantaloupes is different from other fruits and the stomach concentrates on digesting similar types of fruit at a time.

Cherries

Cherries are high in vitamin C, pectin, potassium and soluble fiber. Eating cherries and their juices will help you maintain regular bowel movement when consumed between meals.

Figs

Figs are high in fiber and can be eaten fresh or dried. They are a good source of magnesium, potassium, calcium, iron, Vitamin B6, and Folate. Because they are high in sugar, their stickiness can contribute to tooth decay. So when you eat fresh figs, rinse your mouth out with water afterward.

Eating figs with other fruits high in Vitamin C will increase the absorption of iron. Figs are highly recommended for people who have issues with constipation.

Grapefruits

Grapefruit has a unique type of soluble fiber call galacturonic acid. They are high in vitamin C and potassium. They are a good source of Folate, iron, calcium, beta-carotene, and minerals.

They should not be eaten if you are on blood thinning drugs. When taken with drugs they tend to enhance the effect of the drug or other vitamins taken. Some people are allergic to grapefruit.

Grapes

Grapes are high in pectin and bioflavonoids. They are a good source of iron, potassium and vitamin C. They provide an excellent snack between meals. One problem with them is they are highly treated with pesticides.

Guavas

Guavas are high in lycopene due to its red flesh. It is an excellent source of vitamin C and other nutrients. It is a good source of pectin and other soluble fiber. It contains a good amount of iron and potassium. The outer skin is edible. It can be mixed with other fruit, but eating it alone is better since it will digest faster and provide you with its nutrients quickly.

Lemons are a great source of vitamin C and provide plenty of bioflavonoids and antioxidants. Using the juice of one lemon in the morning with 6+ oz. of water is a great way to help cleanse the liver and the kidney.

Limes like lemons are a great source of vitamin C, bioflavonoids and antioxidants. It also can be used as lime juice in the morning to help the detox process take place in the morning.

Mangos

Mangos are an excellent source of beta-carotene, vitamin C, and fiber. It contains vitamin E, niacin, potassium, and iron. Mangos have been associated with a decrease in breast cancer when eaten regularly. Use it to make morning smoothies.

Nectarines

Nectarines contain plenty of beta-carotene, potassium, vitamin C vitamin A. It's a great source of soluble fiber.

Oranges

Oranges are excellent for vitamin C, beta-carotene, Folate,
thiamin, and potassium. Combine the juice of one or two oranges with one lemon in 8 oz. of water to get your morning going.

Peaches

Peaches are a good source of vitamin A and pectin fiber. It has a useful amount of vitamin C, potassium, antioxidants.

Pears

Pears are a good source of vitamin C, Folate, and fiber. Pears when in season provide for an excellent snack. They tend to ripe fast so they need to be eaten as they turn yellow. Canned pears lose most of their vitamin C value, as do all other fruit that is canned.

Papayas

Papayas contain the protein digestive

enzyme papain. Papain is similar to pepsin, which is the digestive enzyme found in our stomach. They also contain a good amount of vitamin A, beta-carotene, potassium, and vitamin C.

As you can see many of the fruits contain a lot of vitamin C, potassium, beta carotene, antioxidants, bioflavonoids, and fiber. So these are important nutrients, which your body uses during the detoxification process and bodybuilding.

Your body also uses these nutrients to neutralize acids in your cells so that they can continue to function properly and stop the formation of disease.

Eating and drinking the right juices will help to improve your health. As your health improves so will your ability to get a good hard erection. Don't expect results in a few weeks. It took you a long time to diminish your health, so be patient and your health will return.

8: The Best Vegetables That Make You Alkaline

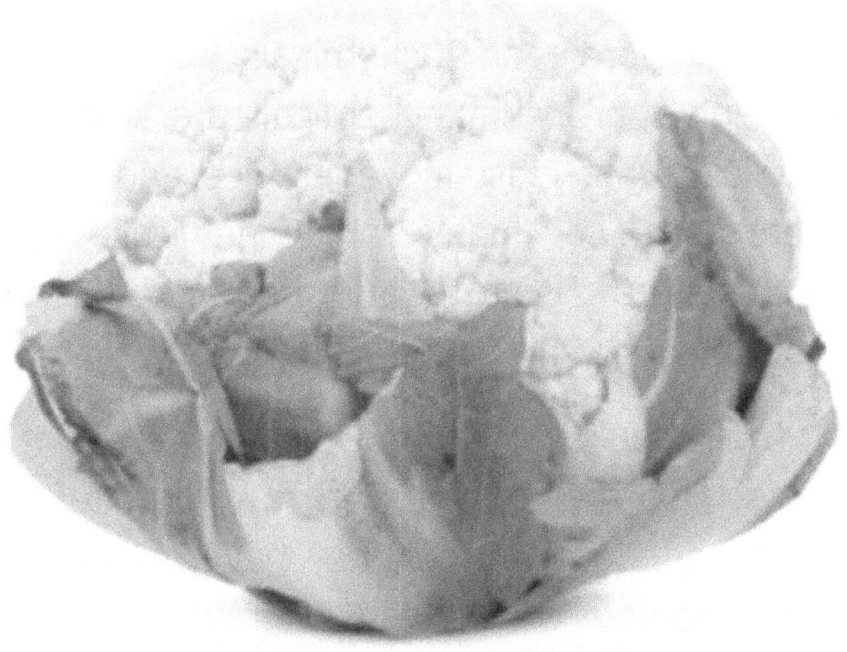

Did you know that there are certain vegetables you should be eating to make your body more alkaline? These vegetables have the chemicals and elements that transform tissues, cells, and organs into an alkaline condition. This is one of their basic functions.

Vegetables and their juices also have

curative powers for preventing and eliminating illness and disease.

Vegetables

The word phytochemicals are used frequently here. Phytochemicals are all of the chemicals that exist in vegetables and fruits. There are so many phytochemicals that scientists have yet to investigate and learn about all of them.

You should be eating vegetables of all colors. Use them, mostly in raw form to get the benefits of the fiber they have, which will help keep your colon clean. In raw form, they contain natural enzymes that help you digest them. And, in raw form, they contain the most vitamins and minerals.

If you cook them in a bit of water and cook them only for up to 4 minutes to keep them firm. Cooking them too long causes them to lose nutrients that you need for your general health.

Always eat vegetables with your main protein or carbohydrate.

This provides the fiber needed to properly digest and move this protein or carbohydrate through your body.

Cooking Vegetables

Vegetables can be stir-fried, steamed, sautéed, or grilled. It is good to eat vegetables in a variety of ways since different nutrients are available based on how they are cooked. By eating vegetable prepared in a different way in a meal, you stand to get the best possible variety of nutrients into your body.

Here are some of the best vegetables to eat raw. There are only a few vegetables that you should not eat raw.

- Bamboo shoots
- Green beans
- Cauliflower

- Collards, Mustard greens
- Chervil
- Chicory
- Corn
- Watercress
- Daikon radish
- Eggplant
- Escarole
- Fennel
- Leek, Shallot
- Lettuce- romaine, butter, red curly
- Mushrooms
- Okra
- Peas
- Bell peppers
- Potato
- Rhubarb
- Rutabaga

- String beans
- Squash, summer, winter, zucchini
- Sweet potato
- Yam

9: Why You Should Drink Vegetable Juices

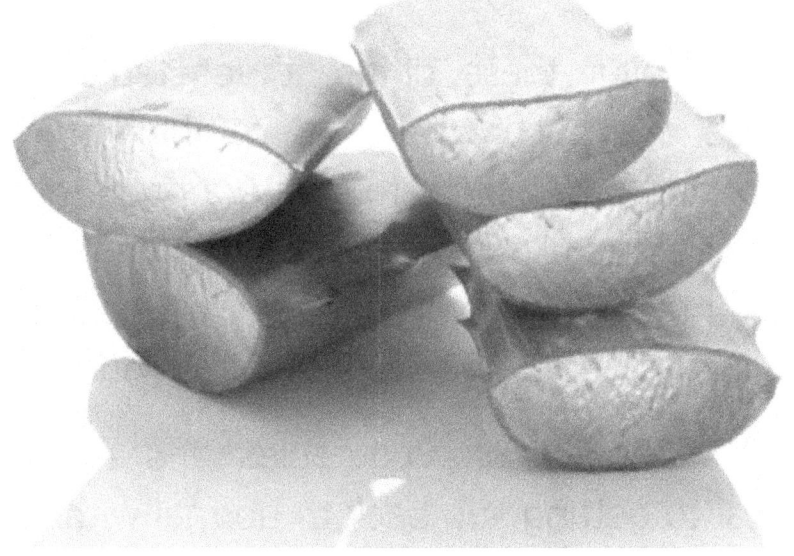

"The continuous and persistent practice of getting the liquid life of fruits and vegetables into the system is one of the secrets of keeping young ..." Dr. Paul Bragg

Creating Health

If you want to regain your health and have strong, hard erections then drinking vegetable and fruit juices is one of the best ways to do this. This produce will move your body to an alkaline condition, remove toxins from your body, calm your nerves, improve your blood circulation, and make your cardiovascular system strong.

Look over these different vegetables and choose one each week and combine it with carrot and other juices to create a drink that is to your taste. Some of these juices don't have a good taste, but consider it medicine and that you don't need to take it the rest of your life.

This chapter on vegetables and fruits is critical to getting you back to normal with your erections. Gaining the best health that you can is the secret to having great sexual performance.

Because fresh fruits and vegetables contain around 70% water, just as our bodies do, they are the perfect food to eat and drink. The water in them provides your body with cleansing and nutritional power.

Fresh vegetable juices have high nutritional, healing, and curing powers. Using vegetable juices as juice therapy has been used throughout the world for centuries to help the body recover from nearly everybody aliment. By separating the juice from its fiber, its minerals and nutrients are suspended in the juice's distilled water.   This allows your body to digest and absorb vegetable juice within minutes as compared with hours when eating the entire vegetable.

The value of fresh vegetable juices lies in the enzymes that they have. Enzymes are the source of life for your body since they provide the vibration or energy for other body chemical reactions to occur.   Enzymes are used in most body chemical reactions and in the digestion of food. They are catalysts that promote chemical action or change without changing their own status or state.

If fruits, vegetables, seeds, or nuts are subject to temperatures from 115F to 120F, their enzymes are destroyed and are no longer active.

Drinking fresh juices especially when you

are sick is one way to recover faster from illness. Vegetable juices digest quicker than then the actual raw vegetable. The digestion of vegetables takes time and energy. The energy to digest the vegetable comes from the vegetable itself. When you are sick, you need to preserve your energy or allow your immune system to use the energy you have to fight off disease. You need to drink more juices when you are sick than when you are not.

Alfalfa Juice

Alfalfa has an array of great vitamins – A, C, K, and Pand over 21 trace and natural minerals. Of course, the actual intensity of the nutrient will depend on the soil it was grown in.

You can use alfalfa juice with any citrus or pineapple juice for allergies. The high alkaline minerals become active in your blood and neutralize any allergens that have activated your allergies.

Alfalfa has chemicals called saponins, which are detergent-like compounds. It is these compounds that can scrub the internal surfaces of your arteries to remove plaque and to prevent its build up. Alfalfa helps you reduce the devastating effects of arteriosclerosis.

Aloe Vera Juice

This juice is used for soothing the bowel area when it is irritated. If you have hemorrhoids it can provide you some relief. Here's how to use it.

There are some aloe vera juice drinks that you can buy at a health-food store. Try them out and see what your results are. If you have the aloe gel, mixture 1-2 tablespoons with 7up or some other carbonated drink. Try different aloe portions until you find one that is palatable.

Artichoke, Jerusalem Juice

This juice is well known for controlling

weight. It does this when this juice is used in a certain way. Artichokes have a high amount of inulin. This is not like insulin but is a carbohydrate that moves quickly into your bloodstream to provide energy for the liver, spleen, and pancreas to help stabilize and normalize your sugar levels. This is a good juice for chronic fatigue syndrome, hypoglycemia, and diabetes. Mix this juice with carrot juice in a one to one mixture.

Mix this juice with equal parts of carrot, alfalfa or beet juice. For a weight loss program, drink this juice through a straw and swish it around in your mouth before swallowing. This helps to reduce your cravings for sweets or junk food.

Asparagus Juice

Asparagus has an alkaloid call Asparagine in high amounts. Asparagine is a non-essential amino acid. Alkaloids are compounds mostly found in plants, and some are good and some are poison. In this case, Asparagine is beneficial for the body. It is an alkaline food and it has been found that the nervous system needs it for proper functioning.

Pure asparagus juice is quite strong, and you should **mix it with carrot juice.** This juice is used as a diuretic and is used for kidney dysfunctions. Its juice is capable of breaking up kidney oxalic stones

It is also good for regulating the prostate and for rheumatism. This juice is also good for people with anemia or who are convalescents

Avocado Juice

Actually, there is no juice that is made from avocados but is it put in a blender with other foods to create an extremely beneficial food. Avocado is considered a complete food because it contains protein, minerals, vitamins, and fatty acids. Avocado has fat in the form of fatty acids – omega 3, omega 6, and omega 9. These fatty acids do not contribute to body fat as many people think, so avocados do not make you fat if you eat them.

Avocados have also been found, in clinical studies, to reduce total cholesterol and at the same time maintain good HDL. A process that is good for the heart and cardiovascular system.

Beet Root Juice

Beetroot resembles turnips. These roots should not be used in summer since it could disturb your sleep or increase your blood pressure. Use them in the winter to keep your body warm and reduce the frequency of colds. It is an excellent tonic for the nervous system and helps to **emulsify and dissolve brain tumors**.

Beet root's sweet juice nourishes and enriches the blood. It's helpful in removing mental dementia and healing wounds. It is a

diuretic, which promotes general health and removes toxins from the body.

You can drink this juice daily if you like. It should be combined with carrot juice – 3 to 8 oz. of beet with 8 oz. of carrot juice. Do not drink beet juice alone, it can cause a cleansing reaction, make you dizzy or cause nausea. If you have just started using this juice, start with a few ounces, and then build up gradually to large amounts.

This juice can be used to build up your red corpuscles. Keep in mind that any juice that is red is good for supporting your blood.

Beets are very high in sodium, so they are good for helping make your body more alkaline. It also has a good percentage of potassium and chlorine. When combined with carrot juice, you get phosphorus, sulfur, and vitamin A.

Beet, Carrot, and Coconut Milk

If you go one step further and add the milk

from the meat of coconuts to carrot and beet juice, you get a combination that is highly alkaline – potassium, sodium, calcium, magnesium, and iron – and also contains phosphorus, sulfur, silicon, and chlorine. This juice is a great bodybuilder and helps to clean out your kidneys and gallbladder.

Beet juice has been shown to be helpful for alcoholism and drug addiction, because of it blood build characteristics. It is able to clear the blood of toxin and to help rebuild the liver, kidney, lungs, heart, and brain, which have been all damaged by the addictive behavior.

Cabbage Juice

Cabbage juice is well known for curing duodenum ulcers, but it has a strong taste. Try combining it with carrot juice for a more palatable drink. It contains a substance called vitamin U, which is not really a vitamin. It is Vitamin U that gives cabbage juice its power to eliminate or cure stomach or duodenal ulcers. Heating cabbage or cabbage juice will destroy the vitamin U and its ability to relieve ulcers.

Drinking cabbage juice regularly can help you reduce nervousness, fear, depression, headaches, restlessness, and trembling, anxiety, and pessimistic views.

Carrot Juice

Carrot juice is the king of juices since it has so many health benefits and can be mixed with other juices to make them more palatable. It rejuvenates the body, produces fresh blood, cleanses the body, produces glowing skin, and provides nutrients for healthy eyes and liver. For those that have a health issue, carrot juice daily is a must to help bring the body back to health.

You can take carrot juice indefinitely and in any reasonable quantity – 1 to 4 pints a day is ok. In his book, N.W. Walker, Doctor of.

Science, Water can undermine your health,

Prescott, Norwalk Press, 1974, recounts his experience with carrot juice,

"There was a time when I first started drinking carrot juice that my skin took on an orange-yellow hue. I discovered that this was due to the cleansing of my liver, which happened to be in VERY bad condition at the time. However, after a few months, the discoloration disappeared and my skin was better and clearer than it had ever been."

If you decide to drink carrot juice daily, there could be a time when you start to feel sick or distressed. Most likely it's not a result of drinking too much juice, but more that you have a lot of body toxins to get rid of.

Celery Juice

This has a high level of potassium. The more potassium you have in your body the more alkaline it is. You can add carrot juice to this juice to make it more palatable. Celery juice is also high in sodium and is considered a sodium food, which is good for your stomach and for making you more alkaline.

If you frequently feel nervous or agitated, try drinking a combination of celery and carrot juice. This combination is good for restoring the function of degenerating nerve sheathing.

The sodium in celery is organic and has nothing to do with the effects of table salt, which has inorganic sodium that the body cannot use. You cannot overdose with natural organic sodium since the body will eliminate the excess organic sodium in your body. However when you eat table salt you can overdose with this sodium, and when you do the kidney has to find a place to store it in your body. This type of storage can lead to edema and high blood pressure because of the water this type of sodium attracts.

Cucumber Juice

You can use cucumber juice to mix with other juices when you cannot use carrot juice.

Cucumber juice is a great source of manganese and is high in vitamin A. If you have a low blood count, then this is the juice for you. Cucumber juice is one of the best diuretics you can use when you need to promote urine.

Dandelion Juice

This juice is high in those minerals that neutralize acids in your body, so use it, if you have an acid body. It is one of the richest foods in magnesium and iron.

Garlic Onion Juice

Garlic belongs to the onion family. Combine this juice with other juices such as parsley, watercress, or spinach.

The combination of onion and garlic provide many complex compounds, but they have 3 important minerals — sulfur, potassium, and germanium.

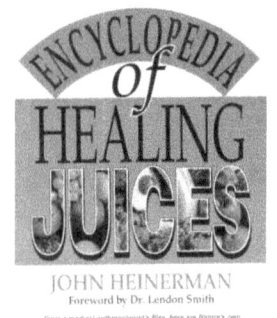

HEINERMAN'S

ENCYCLOPEDIA of HEALING JUICES

JOHN HEINERMAN
Foreword by Dr. Lendon Smith

From a medical anthropologist's files, here are nature's own healing juices for hundreds of today's most common health problems.

In his book, Heinerman, John, Heinerman's Encyclopedia of Healing Juices, Parker Publishing Company, New York,1994, says it all about garlic and onion,

"The final and most important mineral in garlic and onions is sulfur. Doctors, nutritionists, and health writers don't seem to give much attention to this particular trace element.

I've spent almost a decade studying this tremendously important mineral and have discovered in all the research surveyed (including my own) that it is the key to preventing hardening of the arteries, cholesterol buildup in the heart, and to stopping drug-resistant forms of bacteria and fungus.

When combined with other elements such as potassium and germanium in spices like garlic and onion, a powerful trio of chelating agents are formed which keep the heart and liver free of fatty deposits, the immune defenses alert and active, and the condition of the skin healthy and young."

Green Pepper Juice

There are many different green peppers from ones, which are not hot to those that burn your mouth – bell peppers, habanero, jalapeno, and pimento.

It has been found that countries, like Thailand and Mexico, have lower incidents of thrombosis, clots in blood vessels. This may be due to the capsaicin in the peppers they frequently eat.

Green Juices

Using green drinks to improve your health is very important. A green drink can be used

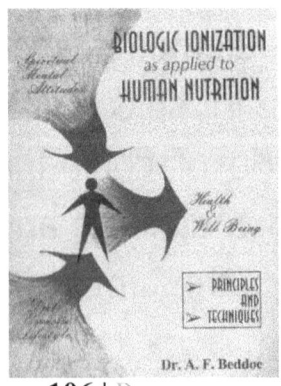

every day. Try to use a green drink at least twice a week. Using liquid chlorophyll is great if you don't have a green drink. Squeeze the juice of one lemon into 1/2 oz. of chlorophyll then add 6 oz. of water. This can be drunk every day first thing in the morning.

Blue Green Manna is another powder you can use. It is high in chlorophyll and enzymes. This Manna is great for regulating the pancreas. You can add a couple of ounces of fresh pineapple, apple, and grape juice to make it more palatable.

Adding a pinch of honey is another way to take a green drink.

In his book, Dr. Beddoe, A.F., Biologic Ionization as Applied to Human Nutrition, S & J Unlimited, Washington, 1994, gives you a recipe for a fresh green drink that you can prepare with a blender,

"Take 2 cups of your favorite juice and place it in a good quality high-speed blender. Add to this a large handful of greens, chosen from the list that follows this paragraph. The amount will vary according to the type of blender used. . . Add as much as can be chopped and blended thoroughly and comfortably, until all greens are well blended for a period of time (3 to 4 minutes) turn off the blender and pour the mixture through a kitchen strainer to remove the pulp. The juice that is left is the green drink."

Use any of the following green leaves:

Bean, dandelion, nasturtium leaves, parsley, wheatgrass, pea pods, romaine lettuce, spinach, beet, carrot tops, celery stalk tops, kale, or any other dark green leaves.

The more chlorophyll you can drink and get into your body the better. Chlorophyll is one of the compounds that green drinks give you. Chlorophyll will slowly chelate, tie up and remove toxic heavy metals out of your body.

Green tea is also an excellent drink since it has one of the highest levels of antioxidants. Green tea is known for gaining excellent cardiovascular health. Drink a cup two times a day.

Prune Juice

Here is the juice that many people use when they have constipation. You can drink a warm glass of prune juice in the morning and it will help you with that day's movements. If you need to get relief from stubborn constipation, then try 2-3 glass in the morning. If you have more than 3 bowel movements a day, you should not drink prune juice. Do not use prune juice for constipation regularly because the more you use it the less effective it becomes.

It can also be used if you have an acid body. It has the minerals potassium, calcium, magnesium, and sodium that will help to neutralize acids in your body.

Radish Juice

At least 1/3 of radish content is potassium and 1/3 is sodium. The radish is also high in iron and magnesium.

Radish juice has a pungent taste and should never be drunk alone. It is best to mix it with carrots, tomatoes, or lemon juices or a combination of all three. It is a great blood purifier and builder and helps blood circulation. It is also useful to rejuvenate and rebuild muscles.

Spinach Juice

Spinach juice should be used by anyone with anemia because of its high iron content. It is also useful in the entire gastrointestinal tract and especially useful for constipation and nervous disorders.

Use Spinach juice as a general or nerve tonic. It is good for sterility, impotence, and fatigue. Spinach is also high in organic oxalic acid and should not be eaten cooked. Eat it raw or juiced to get the natural oxalic acid that your body needs.

Tomato Juice

Tomato juice is to be used in raw form. It

is a blood purifier and stimulates the blood circulation. It cleanses your body of toxins and is a worm killer. Tomatoes help keep your blood alkaline, reduce body acidity, resist diseases, cure liver, and spleen disorders, and also remove chronic fever. Those that have diabetes or prone to nervous conditions should drink tomato juice regularly.

Tomato juice contains lycopene, a potent antioxidant, which has been found to neutralize free radical damage at the cell level. Because of this activity, lycopene has shown to be effective in many types of cancer and cardiovascular diseases.

In cooked form, citric, malic, and oxalic acids become inorganic compounds and have a detrimental effect on your body.

It is best to drink raw tomato juice to get the best benefits from this juice. When this raw juice is drunk with starches or sugar, it acts as an acid food otherwise the body sees it as an alkaline food.

10: Foods That Take Your Manhood Away

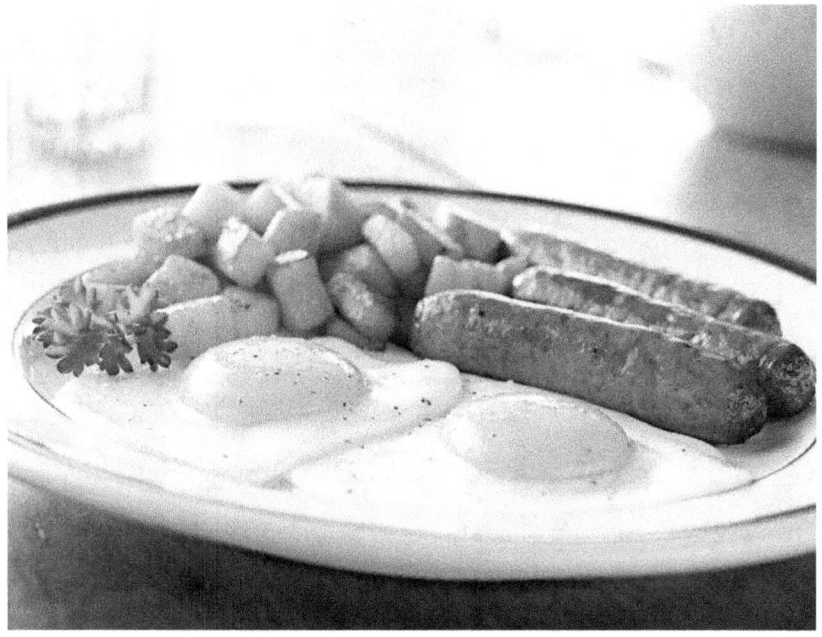

Foods to Avoid Eating

If you smoke, drink alcohol or drink excess coffee, then this program will not work too well for you. When you have these addictions, your body minerals and vitamins will be out of balance and it will be difficult to achieve any state of good health.

If you eat junk food, you need to reduce

the amount you eat. If you limit your use of junk food, you can still maintain some level of health. Here is a way to do it. For 6 days eat healthy food and for 1 day out of 7, you can eat junk food. A healthy body can process junk food out of your body without major harm.

So, here are the foods that you need to stop eating. You don't need to stop eating these foods instantly. Not many people can do this. You need to do this gradually. I know it will be hard to stop eating some of these foods that you have enjoyed, over the years. But later when you have recovered your hardness, you can start eating some of these foods.

The choice is yours and I know you will make the right decision, so here is the list,

White Bread – This is considered junk food since it is void of any vitality for your body. It is hard to digest and causes constipation. Use wheat or a multi-grain bread, but still limit the use of bread.

Chocolate – some chocolate is better than others. Those that have saturated fats such as milk, butter, and sugars are not good for your cardiovascular health. A chocolate that has over 85% pure cocoa has beneficial antioxidants and can fight free radicals that are involved in heart disease.

Try to eliminate the use of **fried foods**. These foods are high in free radical, especially if olive oil or other vegetable or seed oils are used. The best oil to use in cooking is coconut oil, which can withstand higher temperatures before decomposing and forming free radicals.

Fried Fatty foods – fried foods, butter, cheeses,

Foods in packages – all foods in packages or boxes are junk food. They are considered dead food and provide no life force for your body. They take from you because they use up minerals, vitamins, and digestive enzymes during digestion. They contain no fiber so they cause constipation.

Foods with artificial flavors and preservatives - these are non-foods that are super toxic. Your body does not know what to do with them, so it stores them in your body as toxic waste or fat.

Milk, ice cream, hard cheese – these foods cause allergies and cause mucus to form. This mucus coats the colon and other internal surfaces and interferes with the function of that area. Bacteria, viruses, and other pathogens enjoy living in this mucus film, so this makes you more susceptible to colds and flu.

Sodas are the worst drink you can take. They contain plenty of sugar and phosphoric acid.

Table Salt – avoid salt only because it is considered an inorganic matter that contributes to high blood pressure. The more salt you have the less potassium your body retains and this forces your body to hold more water in the areas around your cells and in your cells. The result is higher blood pressure.

If you need to use salt, use sea salt, it has more minerals.

Sugar is the first thing you should pull out of your diet immediately. Eating sugar is responsible for so many serious diseases. It is considered a poison by good health professionals and comes in many dinguses. Here are some forms.

- White sugar (sucrose, brown sugar maple syrup, molasses)
- Fructose
- Glucose
- Maltose
- Lactose
- Corn syrup
- Honey

Eating or drinking any artificial sweetener is even deadlier. The dangers of using these sweeteners are totally underestimated. The liver sees them as a poison.

Smog or Polluted Air

Living in an area of heavy smog or working in an environment that creates polluted air is detrimental to your health. This kind of environment is high in free radicals. Over time, these free radicals will cause damage to your cardiovascular system by creating arterial plaque. This results in less nitric oxide reaching your blood in your genital area and is a major contributor to hardening problems.

11: Nutrients That Change You Into A Real Man

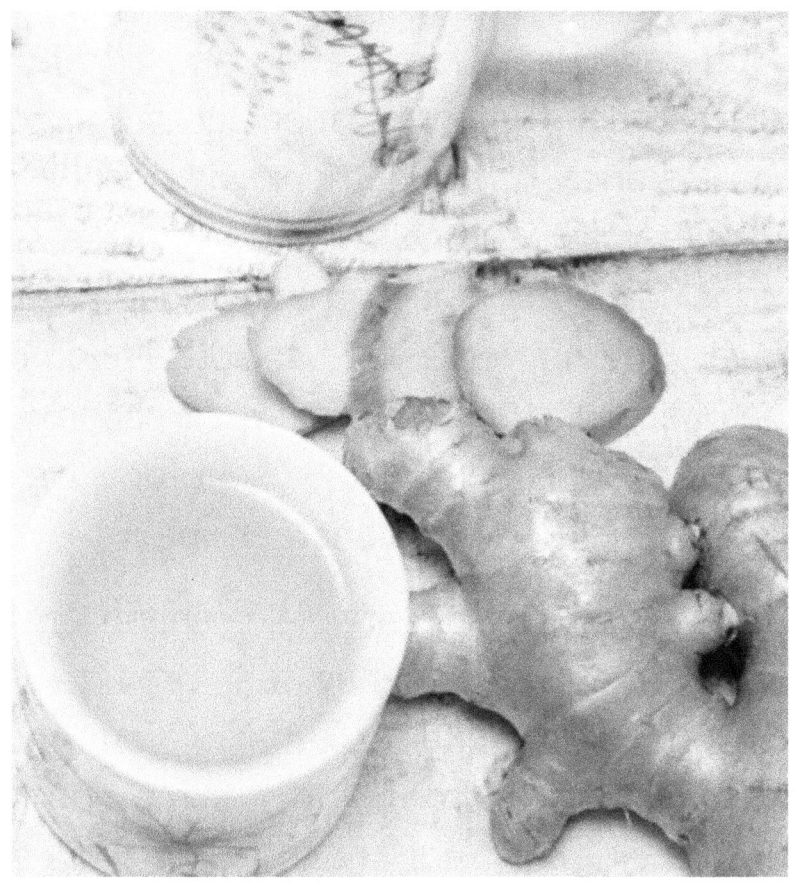

The main reason that you have erection problems is you have poor health, which creates poor blood circulation, insufficient brain nerve signals for nitric oxide stimulation, and poor glandular health in the prostate and other organs. Here are various supplements and herbs that you should start taking daily. Also listed are formulations that contain some of the nutrients you need to take.

You can take a formulation and add other nutrients that the formulation lacks to get a complete array of the nutrient you need. Just pick one or two to get started, but make sure you include L-Arginine and ant-0xidants. You can vary the nutrients you use so that you can experiment with them. But, when choosing a particular supplement to try, use it for 2 weeks before changing over to another one.

There are plenty of male enhancement products that you can buy that promise you just about anything to make you more powerful in the bedroom. Yes, some do work while others may not. Some will work for certain people and they don't work for others. The reason for this is your erectile dysfunction or impotence may be caused by certain conditions that are not similar to others. What this means is that you may need a certain group of nutrients not provided in the enhancement formulation you are trying.

You can look for an enhancement product that might work for you. But, the idea here is to use it for a short time while you work on your whole body to make impotency a thing of the past. Depending on enhancement products long-term is not good practice. You may become addicted to them and would not be able to have an erection without them and they are costly, requiring you to buy them every month.

Here are some of the ingredients that you should look for and that are known to be safe.

Fava Beans

Fava beans have a compound called L-dopa, which has been used to treat Parkinson's disease. L-dopa can also cause you to have an erection. By eating 6-8 oz. of these beans, it could give you enough L-dopa to help give you a better erection. If you know how to sprout seeds, then you can sprout these beans and get even more L-dopa.

Ginkgo Biloba

Ginkgo Biloba has been used to treat high blood pressure and vascular diseases. So it is known to be useful in impotence. In many clinical studies, Ginkgo has been found to increase the blood flow rate in capillaries and end arteries. It helps you create more nitric oxide.

This makes it an ideal herb for treating chronic cerebrovascular insufficiency, diseases of the lower limbs, varicose veins, and post-thrombotic syndrome. It also is effective in decreasing blood clotting.

The action of Ginkgo is to neutralize the effects of free radicals.

These radicals are known for damaging the interior walls of veins and arteries. Damage to these walls causes the buildup of plaque, which then leads to poor blood flow. Poor blood flow is a major problem for those who have problems getting hard. Side effects have been few and relate to gastric disturbances.

Recommend dose is between 120 to 240 mg to be divided into 3 to 4 doses a day. Adjust your dose based on how you feel. If you feel the dose is too high, you can reduce your dose a lower amount.

Ginseng Root Extract

If you want the best Ginseng extract, then you need to get Dr. Schulze's Super Ginseng. This is one of the best formulations you will find. Dr. Schulze has spent years studying how to use roots to create great products. His formulation contains Wild American GINSENG Root, Chinese Ginseng root, Korean Red Ginseng Root, Mongolian Panax Ginseng root and Siberian Eleuthero root.

In a few studies that have been made with ginseng, it was found that some improvement had been made in sexual performance, but not as much as has been seen with other nutrients listed here. However, ginseng is known to help you produce more nitric oxide.

Recommend dose is 1 – 2 droppers full three to four times a day.

Cayenne Tincture and Powder

In her book, Lalitha Thomas, 10 essential herbs, Hohm Press, Arizona, 1992, describes some of the benefits of cayenne,

"Take dose two to four times a day to strengthen the circulatory system, blood vessels and veins; encourage blood to the extremities, and gently dilate capillaries, thereby increasing blood flow and body warmth. This is very good to try for varicose veins, frostbite, and other poor circulation problems. . . Strong, healthy blood circulation to all your body tissues increases your capacity for stamina and recovery from illness."

Clove Tea

Some people have reported that using Clove tea has helped stimulate their sexual organs. It appears to be a sexually stimulating tea. It has effects on the nerves and produces a calming action. This tea helps to create circulation in the penis area.

Oat straw

Oat straw tea has silicon and selenium that will help you recovers your potency. Add two teaspoons to one cup of boiling water and simmer for 15 minutes. Combine this with a good meal plan to get the maximum hardness benefit.

L-Arginine

L-arginine is an amino acid which is absolutely necessary for the creation of nitric oxide. All nitric oxide produced in the penis comes from the presence of L-arginine, a nonessential amino acid. The nitric oxide is produced by the enzyme nitric oxide synthetase acting on L-arginine.

There are two things needed for the production of a good amount of nitric oxide. First, you need a strong neurologic signal, getting sexually excited, to the penis and second, you need a good supply of L-arginine.

The liver can create L-arginine from other amino acids, but if you have a weak liver function or lack a good supply of all the amino acids in your diet, you will not be able to produce enough nitric oxide for a good erection.

Taking a supplement of L-arginine has been proven to create enough nitric oxide in your penis to support the creation of a good erection.

In their book, The Purity Research Department. The

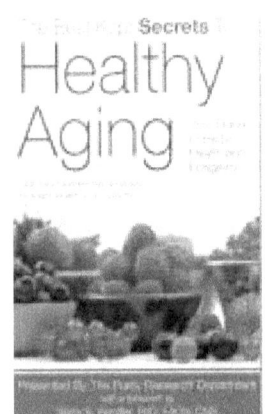

The Best Kept Secrets To Healthy Aging, Purity Products, New York, 2006, they reported,

"For example, 40% of a group of men with erectile

dysfunction to varying degrees responded to 2800 mg of supplemental L-arginine daily for only 2 weeks with 'improved erection' while none responded to weeks of placebo.

Similarly, 6 weeks of daily supplementation with 5000 mg of L-arginine resulted in 'significant improvement in sexual function' in 31% of a group of men with erectile dysfunction, compared to a 12% response to placebo.' Importantly, all of the subjects who responded to L-arginine supplementation exhibited large to increase their rates of NO [nitric oxide] production. It is important to note that a minimum amount of L-arginine must be consumed in order to benefit; men given less than 2000 mg daily have experienced no benefits."

The recommended dose for L-arginine is from 5000 mg to 10,000 mg.

Cnidium

If you have access to Chinese herbs, then the herb to check out is Cnidium. It's a powerful herb that increases nitric oxide levels and improves blood circulation.

Horney Goat

This herb is also a great herb to use for hardness. It will help you produce nitric oxide, testosterone, and reduce your stress and improve your energy. Look for this herb in enhancement formulations.

Pycnogenol

Pycnogenol has been shown to stimulate the production of nitric oxide from L-arginine by increasing the activity of the enzyme nitric oxide synthetase. In a study reported in Journal of Sex and Marital Therapy, Treatment of Erectile Dysfunction with Pycnogenol and L-Arginine, the results showed that with a low dose of L-arginine for a month, men showed no results. Adding a dose of 80 mg of Pycnogenol, 80% of the men showed full restoration of erectile function. The remaining 20% responded when 120 mg of Pycnogenol was added to supplementation.

The recommended dose for Pycnogenol is 200 to 300mg to be taken with a meal or right after a meal.

Korean Red Ginseng

This is a must to be in any enhancement product.   The Chinese, Korea, or Panax ginseng is the most popular. In a study with 45 people with impotency, ginseng was found to improve erectile function and sexual desire.

In an eight week study with 2700mg daily of Korean Red Ginseng and ginseng, erectile function was seen to improve in 60% of the subjects. Other studies have used up to 3000 mg for 12 weeks with no side effects observed and with 66% dramatic improvement reported. The patients had improvements in hardness, penetration, and ejaculation.

Avoid using ginseng, if you have any type of cardiovascular disease. With any signs of cardiovascular disease, consult your doctor before using nutrients that increase your nitric oxide levels.

Pygeum Africanum

Pygeum Africanum is an evergreen tree grown in African and is used for men who have enlarged prostate or prostate problems. If you are over 50, chances are that you have some prostate problems you are not aware of, especially if you have erectile dysfunction. When you have an enlarged prostate, you will have to urinate 2 − 4 times a night. This herb is typically found in a supplement formulation.

African Yohimbe

This herb is a well-known aphrodisiac. Researchers at Stanford Medical School created a powdered derivative called YOHIMBINE, which was shown to be quite effective in tests with lab animals. However, YOHIMBINE is a powerful drug with negative side effects, such as low blood pressure. Using a large amount can kill you, and even small amounts should be used with caution.

You will see Yohimbe bark used in many enhancement products, and this bark is different from the YOHIMBINE that was created at Stanford. Yohimbe bark is considered safer when used in sexual enhancement formulations but still should taken with caution.

Using Yohimbe bark as a single herb is **not recommended**. The reported side effects include increased heart rate, anxiety, increased blood pressure, flushing, headache, and hallucination.

Mura Puama ("potency wood")
Mura Puama is another herb that has been shown in clinical trials to have some effectiveness in improving sexual function.

In studies, no negative effects were seen with this herb. The effects experienced by trail members reported psychological and physical sexual improvement.

Melatonin

Melatonin in clinical studies has been shown to be effective in controlling prostate size. Melatonin is instrumental in the transport and absorption of zinc in the body. We have already noted that the highest levels of zinc in the body are found in semen. The prostate contains large quantities of zinc. If you have low zinc, this will lead to a low sperm count. Melatonin seems to be able to control zinc body levels and thus protect prostate health.

This hormone has been found to fight free radicals just as good as vitamin E. It is one of the chemicals that is able to pass the blood-

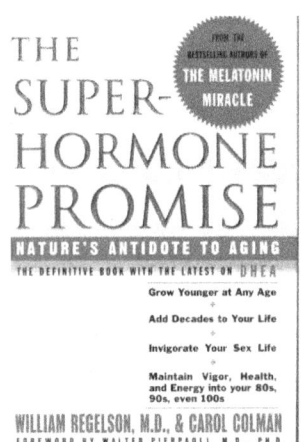

brain barrier and get into your brain to protect it from free radicals. As a result, it has been found effective in keeping your heart healthy, just as vitamin E does.

DHEA

In their book, Regelson, William, M.D., & Colman Carol, The Super Hormone Promise, Simon & Schuster, 1996, talk about how DHEA has helped many people with erectile dysfunction.

"One of the most constantly repeated comments I hear from patients as well as colleagues and friends who are taking DHEA is that it has renewed their interest in sex. Men, particularly, report that it has revived their sexual interest.

Other doctors who prescribe DHEA report that many of their male patients experience an increase in libido and that many older men who did not have morning erections for years suddenly began to experience them after taking DHEA."

In clinical studies, it has been found that as levels of DHEA in the body fall, the incidence of impotency rises. DHEA has also been found to protect against cardiovascular disease. DHEA is converted to testosterone in both men and women. Having adequate testosterone is necessary for having a good libido, sex drive. Just one single supplement like DHEA is not instrumental in beating impotency. To do this requires a combination of all the factors we have been discussing in this book.

Testosterone has many functions in your body. It enhances sex drive, elevates mood, lowers cholesterol and protects against heart disease.

Bee Pollen

Bee pollen has all the vitamins, minerals, amino acids, hormones, enzymes, carbohydrates, essential fatty acids, and trace elements, in the proper proportions, needed for your nutrition. It also contains the gonadotropic hormone, which is similar to the pituitary sex hormone called gonadotropin. This hormone functions as a stimulant for your sex gland.

A good source of bee pollen is Desert Gold from GioLife Pharmaceutical or Montana Pollen Herb Company

Zinc

Zinc is quite important because it is concentrated in the semen. Frequent ejaculation can deplete your zinc stores. Zinc is used not only in semen, but it is used in more enzyme activities than any other mineral. If you are short on zinc, you will suffer a decrease in sexual drive. Just make sure not to take large doses of zinc, since it interferes with the adsorption of copper and calcium. Use the recommended dose below.

Zinc dosage should be around 30 mg.

Essential fatty acids

The best fatty acids to supplement are fish oil. Fish oil provides you with the essential fatty acids in a form that do not require your body to go through too many chemical reactions before you get their benefits.

Vitamin C

Vitamin C helps to strengthen your arteries, veins, and capillaries and to boost testosterone.

B vitamin

Taking B100 vitamin is a good idea. You will need B12, B6, and Folic acid to help neutralize the excess homocysteine that occurs when you eat too much meat. Excess homocysteine in your blood is now associated with the plaque buildup in your artery walls.

Vitamin E

Vitamin E is a major antioxidant substance. It plays a big part in protecting your sperm cells from free-radical damage.

Masulex

Here is a formulation that is made by Enzymatic Therapy. It is a good formulation in that it only contains natural herbs and nutrients. It has many of the herbs listed here. Here is what is in this product.

- Vitamin E
- Liquid Liver Fractions
- Muira Puama
- Damiana
- Proprietary Phytosterol Blend beta-sitosterol, campesterol, and stigmasterol
- Wheat Germ Oil
- Cola Nut
- Panax Ginseng Root
- Saw Palmetto
- Ginkgo

Take a look at this product on the Internet and see if it is something you would like to try.

Green Tea

Using green tea as a drink, capsule, or extract form is a must. Green tea is one of the foods that have the highest antioxidant levels. Because of this, it is very beneficial for the heart and any cardiovascular diseases.

Gerovital GH3 – A General and Sexual Rejuvenator

Here is a great product, but is not sold in the USA, since it was not approved by the FDA when it was first submitted to them. It is used and available throughout Europe and is known as Gerovital H3, GH3® anti-aging supplement.

It appears to be a worthy supplement to use since it is known as an anti-aging and as a sexual enhancement supplement.

To look into this product or buy it, go to

http://www.gh3.co.uk/whybuyhere.htm

Here is a snippet from their website,

"Specific changes included the normalization (either up or down) of blood pressure, the improvement of respiratory functions, increased muscular vigor and basic sex drive, an improvement in arthritic conditions, the disappearance of peptic ulcers, and the normalization of cholesterol levels among many others. The evidence was that the degenerative effects of aging were halted, and in up to 80% of the subjects under scrutiny they even reversed to a significant extent."

It would be best to buy the gold version, which is a pure pharmaceutical grade natural supplement - Gerovital GH3 gold.

12: THE HEART OF A REAL MAN, THE KEY TO HARDNESS

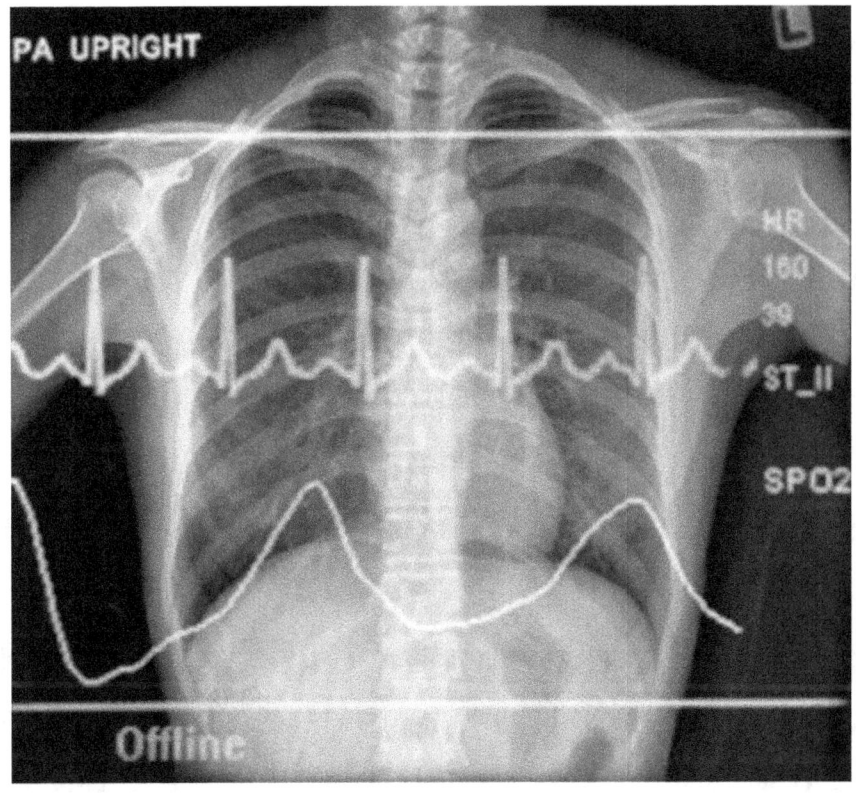

Having erectile dysfunction is an issue of proper blood circulation and nitric oxide release. This issue is an indication of the poor health of your cardiovascular system. Close attention must be paid to this correlation. In this chapter, you will find information that will help you strengthen your heart and cardiovascular system.

Melatonin

Melatonin is not only used to get a better sleep. Here is a secret that doctors in the know keep to themselves. There is no money in recommending Melatonin to lower high blood pressure, control cholesterol levels, protect against stress, and prevent heart attacks and stroke. This is exactly what Melatonin can do.

One of the main hormones of the pineal gland is melatonin. There is a close relationship between the function of the pineal gland and the heart. In studies, melatonin was found to normalize cholesterol in high-cholesterol diets. It was also found that in people with normal cholesterol levels melatonin did not change their cholesterol levels.

There are indications that melatonin

protects against high blood pressure. When you sleep, your body puts out melatonin and at that time, your heart rate slows and blood pressure drops. As soon as you wake, there is a sharp rise in blood pressure. It has been noted that during the hours of 6 am to 9 am is when most heart attacks occur.

Melatonin has also been found to control the production of corticosteroids from the adrenal gland. In excess, corticosteroids released in a fight or flight condition has been found to be damaging to your heart.

Dose recommended for Melatonin can range from 1 mg to 10 mg. An average dose is around 3 to 5 mg. You can experiment with different doses when you go to sleep. If you get a headache, back off on the dose the next night. Using melatonin regularly can help you maintain better heart health and keep your arteries from becoming clogged with calcium deposits as you age.

The body systems that regulate high blood pressure include various body organs, hormones, and nerve impulses. When things change in this system, high blood pressure can occur. As mentioned before look at your stress, your use of salt, drugs, excess weight, smoking, or alcohol and make some effort to reduce their use.

Cholesterol

Here's what The Sherpa had to say about cholesterol in one of his email newsletter, Natural Health Sherpa LLC, Wilmington, NC,

"Hello, Sherpa Follower,

Don't let the hype fool you.

Your cholesterol levels have nothing to do with your risk for heart disease.

This is not just an outrageous claim. Its proven fact backed up by peer-reviewed scientific studies.1-3

The most detailed of them all, the Framingham Heart Study, looked at risk factors for heart disease in over 5,000 men and women over their lifetimes. It clearly showed that 80 percent of people who go on to have a coronary artery disease have the same total blood cholesterol values as those who don't go on to have heart problems.4.

Experts now realize that chemical transformation of LDL by free radical attack is the first, necessary step for dangerous plaque buildup in your arteries - and the real indicator of your risk for heart attack and stroke."

In this book, we focused on LDL cholesterol as the culprit for heart attacks or cardiovascular disease and HDL as the powerful agent to prevent attacks. All food, exercise, antioxidants, and nutrients focused on lowering LDL and increasing HDL.

Here are the main cholesterol levels you need to be concerned with:

- Total Cholesterol, which is a combination of LDL-C AND LDC-C - try for less than 100 mg/dl.

- Low-density lipoprotein, LDL or bad cholesterol - try for less than 160 mg/dl.

- High-density lipoprotein, HDL, Good Cholesterol - try for less than 35 mg/dl.

High Blood Pressure

High blood pressure is a risk factor for heart attack, stroke, loss of vision, and kidney disease. High blood pressure is usually caused by plaque buildup along your artery walls, kidney disease or the lack of potassium. In my Kindle e-book called, _Potassium Health Secrets Revealed_, you can get all the information on how to improve your health using potassium.

Exercise

Exercise is important in lowering high blood pressure. So, you
need to develop some type of exercise that can work on your heart.A good program to use is called PACE. More information on this

program will be provided in the chapter on exercise.

Poor Circulation

Poor blood circulation is directly associated with impotence. This, in turn, is caused by atherosclerosis, hardening of the arteries, where the arteries get narrower, due to plaque buildup along the artery walls. Atherosclerosis is a disease that does not happen suddenly. It occurs slowly over the years of your life.

Good blood circulation produces a hard erection whereas poor blood circulation produces a weak erection or no erection at all.

Footbaths

Foot baths are under-utilized natural processes that can bring herbal nutrients into your body through your soles in an easy and safe way. For high blood pressure or for poor circulation, you can use herbs that directly influence a change in those conditions. You can buy a foot bath that heats the water and has some massage jets. Here's how to use the foot bath for improving your blood circulation.

Buy the following herbs leaves, roots or powders and create an infusion by putting a full tablespoon of these dry herbs into boiling water. Turn down the heat and simmer the infusion for 15-20 minutes. Place herbs through a strainer to capture the leaves or roots. Put hot water into your foot bath, so you don't have to wait for it to heat up. Now, add the herbal infusion. When the water temperature is usable, put your feet in with the heater and bubbler on. Keep your feet in the foot bath from 15 to 20 minutes.

Here are some herbs that you can use for poor circulation and high blood pressure. Always include cut up pieces of garlic in your herb infusion and a pinch of cayenne. You will have to test on how much cayenne to put in the infusion. But, start with a very small amount, since it is a very powerful herb and can overheat your feet fast. You don't have to use cayenne if it becomes too uncomfortable.

Buy these loose herbs in 1 to 2 oz. Then mix them all together. Take one full tablespoon of this mixture to create your infusion.

- Hawthorne leaf
- Ginseng root of different kinds
- Licorice root
- Parsley
- Ginger root
- Butcher's broom
- Kelp
- Ginkgo Biloba
- Garlic
- Oatstraw
- Yarrow
- Dandelion root

If you can't find all of these herbs, it's ok. Just use the ones that you can find.

Warning: if you are pregnant, has a pacemaker, suffers from diabetes, phlebitis and/or thrombosis, are at an increased risk of developing blood clots, or have pins/screws/artificial joints or other medical devices implanted in your body, then you should consult with a physician before using a footbath as described above.

13: EXERCISES THAT INCREASE YOUR MALE PERFORMANCE

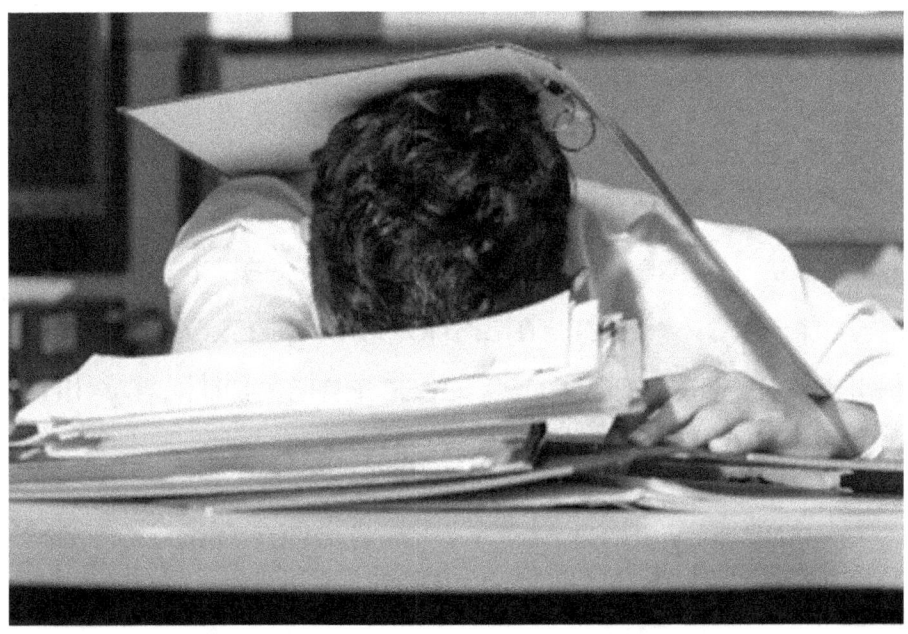

So why is it important to do exercise to eliminate erectile dysfunction? The main reason is that when you exercise you create more nitric oxide. When blood flows faster through your arteries, it stimulates the cells in the artery walls to produce nitric oxide. In previous chapters, you saw that nitric oxide is one of the major processes that control how hard your penis gets. For that reason, you need to do some form of exercise.

Exercise research studies have found that the more physically fit a man is the better his sexuality.

PACE® is the first and only program conceived, designed, tested and proven to achieve this most important of all fitness goals. It does this for you by measuring where you are, then making progressive, small, incremental changes over time. Little by little you advance to the next level.

The key is to start with a brief exertion that is comfortable for you at your current capacity. It's not so important how hard you exert yourself today. It's that little bit that you do next week, which you didn't do this week. This is the element of progressivity. By changing your program through time, you work with your metabolism and your inborn adaptive response to coach your body to change.

Learn Progression with This Easy 10-Minute PACE® Program

Here's a simple program to use progressivity in the right direction. In this 10-minute program below, you're going to focus on gradually increasing the challenge, each time you exercise.

The exercise you do is what you can do at home with any equipment you might have. It can be a stationary bicycle, a treadmill, or a rebounder. You can even run in place, or if you belong to a gym, you can use their equipment.

Exertion   Recovery   Exertion   Recovery   Exertion Recovery

Week	Warm-ups	Set 1	Set 2	Set 3
1	*2 min	**5 min	***3 min	
2	1 min	3 min	2 min	3 min

3	1 min	2 min	2 min	2 min
	2 min	2 min	2 min	
4	1 min	1 min	2 min	1 min	2 min
	1 min	2 min		

*Warm is the time you will stretch and get ready to exercise

**Exertion is the time you do the exercise

***Recovery is the time where you slow down your exercise so you can recover your heart rate to a normal beat.

Notice the progressivity of this workout. Over time, the duration of each exertion period decreases. This progressivity in the right direction toward maximal capacity is the heart of PACE®.

Here's how it works...

During week 1, you're going to take it easy and just do one warm-up for 2 minutes and then one exercise set at a low to moderate intensity for 5 minutes. Just do what feels comfortable. If you are out of shape, it's okay. You can just start walking. Then you will recover for 3 minutes.

Try and do these 10-minute interval exercises at least three times during the first week. But each time you do it, slightly increase the intensity level. By the end of the first week, you should feel like you've given yourself a slight challenge.

Changing The Exercise Intensity

Keep in mind that how you adjust the intensity will depend on what exercise equipment you're using. If you're on a stationary bike, increase the level on the control panel so it becomes harder to pedal. If you're on an elliptical, boost the incline so it's harder to run, etc.

During week 2, you'll add another exercise set. But the duration of your exertion periods will decrease. After a quick warm-up, you'll do a 3-minute exertion period and a 2-minute cooldown. As you start, notice how fast you're going and how long it takes for your heart and lungs to meet the challenge.

When 3 minutes is up, begin your recovery. If you need to stop, that's okay. Otherwise, your recovery period should be a slow, easy pace. If you're on an elliptical machine, for example, you should slow down so you feel like you're walking.

During each recovery period, you should focus on your heart rate, so if you start to pant, it is okay. Feel your lungs quickly fill up and release. Allow your body to come back to a state of rest. This is strengthening your heart and lungs.

During week 3, you'll start with a quick warm up and then a 2-minute exertion period. But this time, increase the intensity to give yourself more of a challenge.

When 2 minutes is up, begin your recovery. Repeat this exercise process 2 more times. During week 3, try and repeat this workout 3 or 4 times.

When you hit week 4, you're going to do 3 exercise sets as in week 3. Except for this time, you're going to reduce the exertion periods to just 1 minute each, followed by 2-minute recovery periods.

Apply the same principles. Take your warm-up at a low to

moderate intensity. Then turn up the intensity when you start your first exertion period.

Remember, don't stress yourself. As you decrease the exertion duration, you turn up the intensity. And by decreasing the duration, it will actually feel easier as the 4 weeks progress. Part of the PACE® program is realizing that real progress can be made in just minutes a day.

To get the full Pace program go to the Internet to find it. It is an excellent way to exercise for a short time and still get the benefits of losing weight and strengthening your heart.

14: Natural Body Cycles

That Help You Become A Man

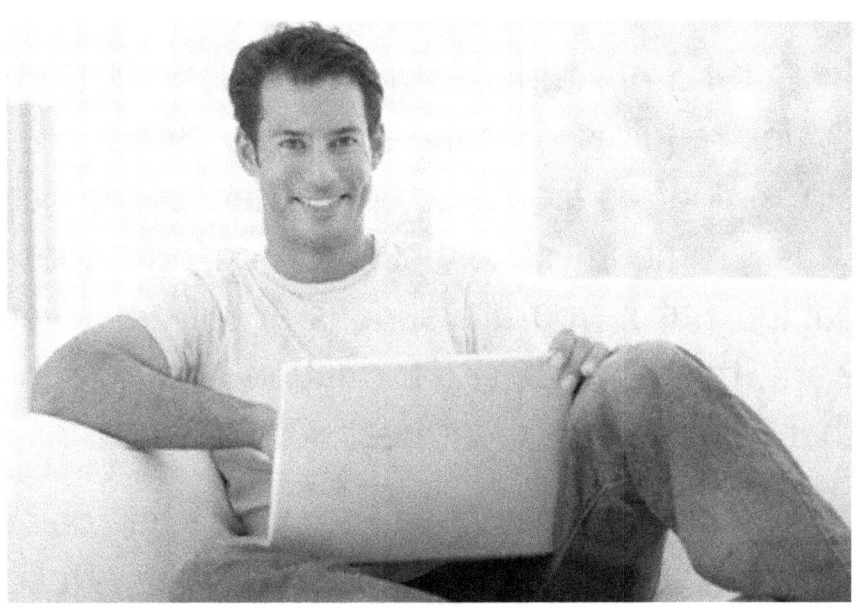

Natural Body Cycles

Most of you are looking for ways to get rid of constipation, improve your health, or lose weight. Here's some information that will help you achieve these results. It's called "Using the Natural Body Cycles" for achieving maximum health.

By learning how to assist your "Natural Body Cycles", you will be in tune with what your body is doing to eliminate fecal matter from the colon and toxic wastes from your lymph liquid and blood.

Getting in tune with your Natural Body Cycles requires a change in the way you eat. Since all of us are addicted to the way we eat, it is, sometimes, difficult to change these habits. But if you are serious about what you want, this is the best information I have found that will give you great health.

Using this method to gain better colon health, you may experience side effects because you will be eliminating more body toxins and body wastes. The side effects maybe headaches, stomach upsets, body pain, or similar types of symptoms. These conditions will not last and will disappear as you get rid of more toxins. So if you experience these side effects, don't let them stop you from moving forward on this eating pattern.

Here are the 3 natural body cycles:

Cycle 1 time period: 4 am to noon

This cycle is the time where your body is eliminating toxins, acids, wastes, and derby by urine, bowel movements, and other secretions. Most people interfere with this cycle, since they are unaware of it, causing constipation and various detrimental illnesses.

Cycle 2 time period: noon to 8 pm

This is the time when your body should be taking in food and digesting it. By eating the right kind of food, you help your digestive process in your stomach and small intestine.

Cycle 3 time period: 8 pm to 4 am

This is the time your body is absorbing and using the food you have eaten from noon to 8 pm.

The First Body Cycle

During the elimination cycle, 4 am a.m. to noon, eat and drink only fruits and their juices or drink vegetable juices.

For breakfast, eat a bowl of fruit or have a fruit smoothie made with apple juice, banana, and fruits in season. Before noontime eat fruits as a snack. Forty-five minutes before noon eat your last fruit. You can eat and drink all the fruits and juices you want up to noontime.

Fruits are made by nature and are a perfect food. They contain the right balance of nutrients with about 70% distilled water. You gain enormous benefits from eating fruits especially if you eat the outer skin. Eat them without cooking them. They are easy to digest and absorb and do not stress your colon. They activate peristaltic action in your colon and help you have a bowel movement.

Here are some of the fruits to eat:

Apples

Apricots

Avocados

Bananas

Blueberries

Boysenberries

Cantaloupes

Cherries

Figs and dates

Grapes

Grapes

Lemons

Nectarines

Oranges

Papayas

Peaches

Pears

Persimmons

Plums

Prunes

Raspberries

Strawberries

Watermelons

Eat all melons together and not with other fruit and wait 1/2 hour before eating other fruits. Melons require specific enzymes to be digested in the stomach, so other fruit eaten with melons will just sit in your stomach, waiting to be digested and can cause gas and an acid stomach.

By eating fruits during body cycle 1 you are assisting your body's elimination cycle. This helps your body to have bowel movements and eliminate toxins and acids from your body and blood. It is these toxins and acids that make you sick, overweight, constipated.

Eating solid food for breakfast – eggs potatoes, rice, meat, cereal, milk, and so on, the typical breakfast, interferes with your body's elimination cycle and eventually leads to sickness and excess weight. It takes over 3 hours to digest heavy and solid food. The food you should be eating in the morning should digest quickly to help activate peristaltic colon action to help you have a bowel movement and to continue your body's detoxification process.

Heavy food slows down the elimination of toxins from your body and this causes chime to remain in your colon and toxins to remain in your body. These toxins then get stored in your body as fat and acids. Acids are the main cause of most illnesses, so you want to have an alkaline body. Fruits and vegetables neutralize acids and give you an alkaline body. An alkaline body is the healthiest body condition you can have.

It takes ½ to 1 hour or so to digest fruits and fruit juices. Because of this, they help to cleanse your body of waste during the time from 4 am to noontime. Fruits are 70% water, just like your body, and this gives them the cleansing action they have and that your body needs.

So if you are not already having fruit and fruit vegetable juices for breakfast and snacks, start slowing changing your habits, if you want to lose weight and feel better.

Now, one other thing, don't eat fruits and juices with your lunch or dinner meals. Wait for at least 1 to 1 ½ hours before eating fruit snacks.

The Second Natural Body Cycle
Here is the second body cycle and it occurs from noon to 8 pm.

This is the time when your body should be taking in food and digesting it. During this period it is time to eat solid food. What you eat has to be in alignment with what your stomach can do.

Here's how your stomach works. In general, it can only digest one solid food at a time.

A solid food is one that does not contain 70% water, like fruits and vegetables do, and whose water has been eliminated by heat or other food processes, in other words, cooked.

Your stomach can only work on one solid food at a time, so your lunch and dinner should only have one solid food. A lunch can consist of chicken and a green salad, fish and a green salad, tuna and a green salad, shrimp and a green salad, beef and a green salad.

Mixing a protein meal with carbohydrates is giving the stomach two solid foods at the same time, which require different concentrations of digestive juices.

Giving the stomach more than it can handle interrupts the elimination cycle 1 and reduces the energy that you need for the elimination cycle.

Any eating habit that disrupts cycle 2, the eating and digestion cycle, affects the other cycles. Here's how you can help your body's cycle 2 to be more effective.

1. Eat only one solid food with vegetables during lunch or dinner. Lunch can be one meat or seafood with a fresh vegetable salad.

2. Limit the amount of water you drink during meals. Excess water will dilute your digestive acids and slow down your digestion. Avoid drinking sodas, tea or other drinks during your meals. If you need to clear your dry throat, use room temperature water. Cold liquids will slow down your digestive processes.

3. Eating meals with more than one solid food such as meat and potatoes, chicken and rice, fish and rice, chicken and noodles, eggs and toast, cheese and bread will diminish the energy you need during the elimination cycle

4. It is permissible to eat beef and chicken at the same time but not chicken and eggs or beef and nuts or chicken and beans. Eat the same type of protein at the same time but do not mix different proteins.

5. It's ok to eat different types of carbohydrates at the same time, with a salad, but not with protein, since carbohydrates digest easier than protein.

Eating a protein and a carbohydrate at the same time sets the stage for severe illness later in life. A protein requires acid for digestion, and a carbohydrate requires alkaline juices for digestion. This combination produces acid juices and alkaline juices at the same time. This combination produces water, which creates digestive juices that cannot fully digest either type of food.

In this case, the body produces more acid and more alkaline juices, which again are neutralized. The cycle continues until the food in your stomach starts to putrefy and ferment causing gas and acids. The gas causes belching and the combination gas and acids can lead to acid reflux.

As food turns into acids because of putrefaction and the fermentation process, this acid food spoils all of the food in your stomach, causing undigested food to backflow up your esophagus and flow prematurely into your small intestine.

Food that is partially undigested becomes acidic, which affect the health of your colon and cause constipation. When these acids are absorbed into your body they are converted into fat and stored as toxins your body.

In many cases, the fermentation of food results in the production of alcohol and is similar to a person who drinks alcohol. There have been cases where people have been arrested for drunk driving and have never drunk in their life, and they wonder why they had a high blood-alcohol level.

Eating the right combination of foods at meal time helps to preserve your energy for the elimination cycle and prevents you from creating spoiled food in your stomach that is converted to acid waste. It is this acid waste that results in illness and fat. This is the reason most people as they age come down with various illnesses that terminate their lives early or gain excessive weight.

Again, the three body cycles are:

Cycle 1 time period: 4 am to noon - This cycle is the time where your body is eliminating toxins, acids, wastes, and derby by urine, bowel movements, sweat, mucus, and other secretions.

Cycle 2 time period: noon to 8 pm - This is the time when your body should be taking in food and digesting.

Cycle 3 time period: 8 pm to 4 am - This is the assimilation period.

The Third Body Cycle

The third body cycle is the assimilation cycle and is from 8 pm to 4 am. This is the time the food you have eaten during the day is assimilated, absorbed and distributed throughout your body through your blood. It is the time where digested food moves into the colon as chime and is stored there for elimination. And, you should be eliminating this chime or fecal matter, when you wake up or during the morning, up to noon.

Food eaten during the second cycle, noon to 8 pm that was combined and eaten properly will digest within three hours, whereas food not combined properly, a meal consisting of protein and carbohydrates will take up to 8 hours to pass through the stomach. During this time, your food will putrefy and ferment and become acidic. Under these conditions, you will not get many nutrients from that meal.

So, eat your last meal by 6-7 pm, so that your food digests in your stomach by the time you go to bed. Three hours later, your food will have moved into your small intestine where it is ready for assimilation.

When you go to bed three hours after your last meal, the next 6 hours, until 4 am, your body will be absorbing the food you have eaten the previous day and moving waste into your colon.

Remember, anything you do differently than what these cycles call for will disrupt them and cause them to become extended. When this happens, your food turns into acid, you don't absorb the value of your food, you lose energy and become tired, and over time, you gain weight and create constipation and serious illnesses.

Have you ever noticed how everyone you know eventually comes down with some sickness, which requires surgery or doctor's drugs? Think about it. Is this what you want to happen to you? Just start changing your eating habits slowly and as time passes you will be doing more and more of what your body's natural cycles need.

15: How To Cleanse Your Colon For Sexual Health

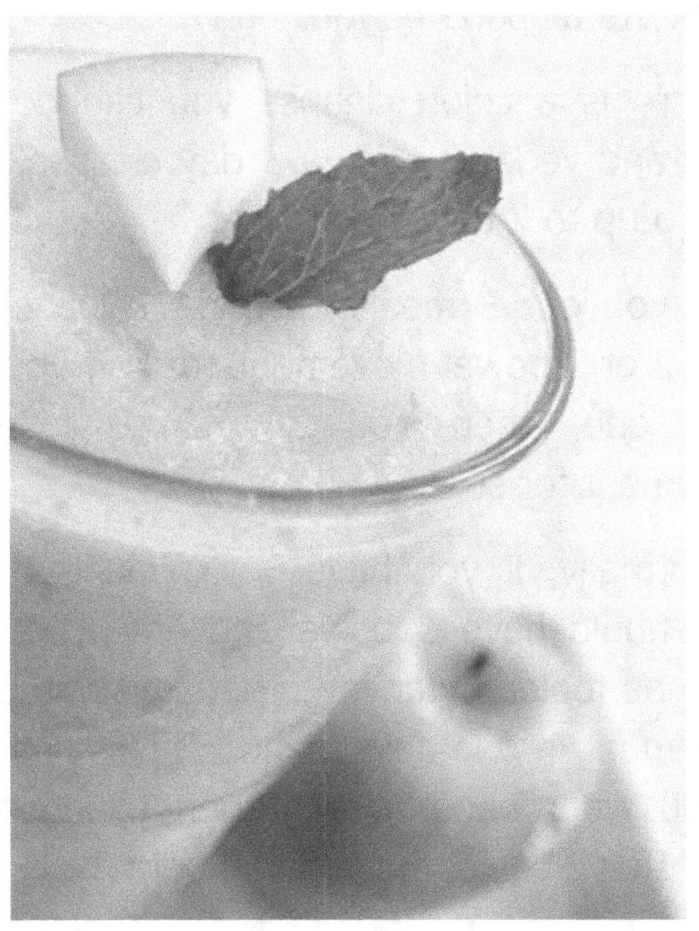

In any health program, the first thing you need to do is a colon cleanse. Once you do this, whatever health program you start, you will get the maximum benefits of the new program. To keep good health, you need to make sure you have regular bowel movements. If you are not regular, you will have a toxic colon that will be supplying toxicity to all parts of your body.

Here is a colon cleanse you can do with fruits and vegetable for a 3 day cleanse. You can go up to 7 days if you like.

If you eat 3 meals each day, you should have 2 or 3 bowel movements day. If you only have one, then you are short 1 bowel movement for sure.

Normally, if you have 3 full meals a day, you should have 3 bowel movements a day. Don't be fooled by anyone that says one bowel movement in two days is ok. This is not true. If you want good health, then you need to have 1 or 2 bowel movements per day.

If you want to learn how to keep regular using natural remedies then you can check out my e-book called,

"Constipation Natural Cures" Look for it on Google.

So let's get started.

To get your bowels moving like they should, you need to clean out what is in your colon right now. So the first day is for cleaning out your colon. The next two days is for cleaning the colon and to detoxify the body.

Doing a colon cleanse of a minimum of three days is the best way to start cleaning out your colon, to detoxify the blood, and rejuvenate your body. Just doing a cleanse for three days is not a cure-all, and it will require more work on your part by starting to eat more natural foods and using the natural body cycles.

I consider this a mini-fruit juice cleanse. This is to start your body detoxifying. You can do this juice fast once a month for 2-3 days, but leave out the prune juice or just use the prune juice every other month and just drink the juices for 2-3 days. This gives your stomach, small and large intestine and liver a rest and a chance to rejuvenate.

Doing a juice cleanse can give you some side effects, where you are nausea or slightly sick. Not everyone will get these effects.

This three-day colon cleansing is outlined in my "<u>Colon And Blood Cleansing Diet</u>." In kindle form. But the information you have here is sufficient to do the 3 days cleanse.

In her extensive book, Cooking For Healthy Healing, 1991, Linda Rector-page, N.D., Ph.D., talks about what a fast does,

"Fasting works by self-digestion. During a cleanse, the body in its infinite wisdom, will decompose and burn only the substances and tissue that are damaged, diseased, or unneeded, such as abscesses, tumors, excess fat deposits, and congestive wastes. Even a relatively short fast can accelerate elimination from the liver, kidneys, lungs, and skin, often causing dramatic changes as masses of accumulated waste is expelled. Live foods and juices can literally pick up dead matter from the body and carry it away."

The day before the fast

The day before the fast, eat a large salad and two apples. This will give you plenty of fiber to scrub the walls of your colon as you move fecal matter out of your colon the following day.

The first day of colon cleanse

Do this cleanse on a Saturday, Sunday or any other day that you don't have to go anywhere. You may be going to the bathroom all day, and at times you need to be there quick. I have done this cleanse even during a workday.

Buy the following items.

- Organic apple juice – one gallon
- Organic apples – 6 for one day
- Organic prune juice – one quart

When you first wake up in the morning, drink,

8 oz. of prune juice

- 10 minutes later drink another 8oz of prune juice
- 10 minutes later again drink another 8 oz. of prune juice
- wait 20 minutes then drink 8 oz. of apple juice
- wait 30 minutes then drink another 8 oz. of apple juice

If you haven't sped to the bathroom yet, you will in a little while.

Now you will drink 8 oz. of apple juice every hour, until the end of the day. You can stop drinking apple juice around 5 pm.

During the day, you can eat three apples in the morning and three apples in the evening.

This process will clean out any fecal matter that has been sitting your colon for days and gets you ready for the next step.

The second way to start the colon cleanse

Another way to start a colon cleanse is to use a product that is called "Oxy-Powder." This product is in capsules and is used for 30 days. Simply by taking capsules every day, you will clean out your colon and any build up along your colon walls.

This is a very effective product and will send you to the bathroom frequently as it cleanses out your colon. Start this cleanse on a Saturday so you can have Saturday and Sunday free to start cleaning. For a gentle cleanse you can start with about 4 Oxy-Powder capsules. Take the capsules the night before you start your cleanse. For a more powerful start on your cleanse take 6 to 8 capsules. But be ready during the day to go to the bathroom frequently.

The first day of the cleanse start drinking and eating apple juice or any other fruit or juice that you like all day.

After two days of intense cleaning, you can back off on Oxypowder and continue to take a lower capsule dose of 2 to 3 capsule per day.

You can get Oxy-Powder on the Internet.

The second day of the colon cleanse
During the second day, you can drink different kinds of juice and eat 2-6 apples. You can drink any kind of juice be it fruit or vegetable. A combination of fruit and vegetable juice is good.

The third day of the colon cleanse

The third day is like the second day where you can drink different kinds of juice and eat 2-6 apples or other fruit. You can drink any kind of juice be it fruit or vegetable. A combination of fruit and vegetable juice is good. If you like you can eat some steamed vegetables.

Fourth Day, after the fast, is done

After you have finished your three-day fast, start eating soft foods to gently adjust your system to food. Here are some of the foods you can eat on the fourth day out of your fast,

- Baked potato
- Fruit salad
- Fruit smoothie
- Light soup
- Oatmeal, multigrain cereal with banana
- Salad
- Natural Yogurt

Fifty Day

On the fifty day start using the ideas given here on eating a healthy diet. You can continue to use Oxypowder at 2 capsules every night for the rest of the month. Oxypowder is not a laxative, even though it made your stools runny the first days of cleansing. So you don't have to worry about being addicted to this product.

16: A System To Eliminate Erectile Dysfunction

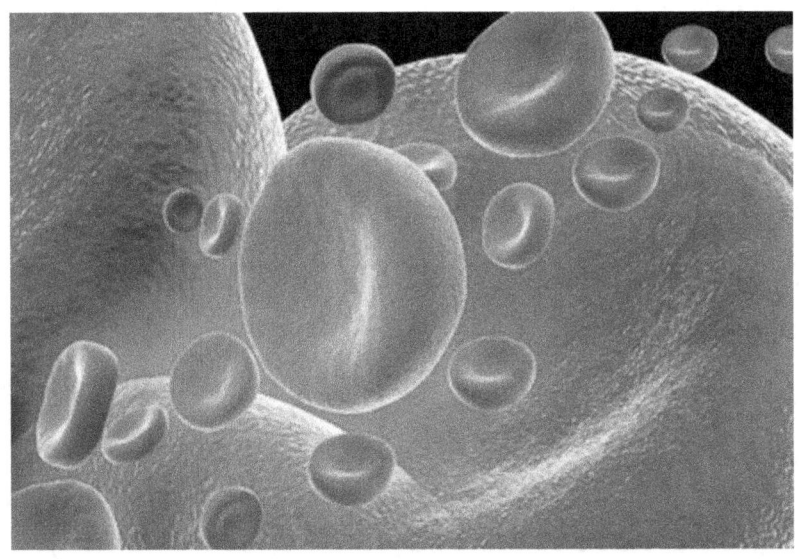

One thing to think about is the old saying, "If you don't use it, you lose it." So, start this hardness recovery program right away. The longer you wait, the more difficult it will be to recover your hardness.

I have given you a lot of information and it can be confusing as to where to start and what to do. There are many directions you go in to work on your erectile issue. And what

I'm about to suggest is just one direction. You can create your own plan using the information that I have given you here. But here is a summary of what has been said in this book.

If you have been having problems getting an erection for a few times, this is not erectile dysfunction. For some reason, you have lost confidence in producing a strong and hard erection, and that will pass. But, if it continues then, you can do something about it, using this information.

The causes of impotence are varied, but some of the areas that you need to work on are:

1. Eliminate bad habits that create a cardiovascular disease

2. Create an alkaline body for normal health and to eliminate illness

3. Stimulate your brain to improve your libido or sexual desire

4. Improve your blood circulation to improve the flow of blood to your penis

5. Increase Your nitric oxide to promote hardness

6. Improve nerve function to stimulate your sexual centers

7. Improve hormonal balance to normalize your sexual secretions

Bad habits

I have listed which bad habits you need to change or minimize. These include smoking, using medical drugs, using over-the-counter remedies, drinking alcohol, and a few others. If you are not able to make these changes then, this health program will not be as effective.

The reason you have hardness problems is because of the lifestyle you are living and if you want to improve your hardness, then you need to make some drastic changes.

You don't have to make these changes all of a sudden. You need to withdraw from them slowly, by decreasing your dependence on them weekly and by reducing the quantity you use.

Alkaline body

You need to change your body condition from acid to alkaline. Having an acid body is a major reason why some many people are sick with a variety of deadly diseases. You can recover your health by creating an alkaline body.

First, you need to do is a three day cleanse as outlined in a previous chapter. This will clean out your colon and cleanse your blood. This will make your body more alkaline and give you a great start for what follows next.

Next, you need to follow the body cycles. The eating patterns suggested here are so that you can help your body to continue to eliminate toxins normally. These toxins make your body malfunction and keep your body acidic.

Next, you need to incorporate better eating habits by eating the protein, fruit and vegetable juices, fruits, and vegetables. Use the juices daily and discover which ones you like and which one makes you feel better.

This is the way to get an alkaline body, which will help you improve your cardiovascular, nerve function, hormonal balance, and overall health. Eating good protein helps to rebuild those weak muscles throughout your body, including your penis.

Brain Stimulus, Nitric Oxide, Blood Circulation

Now it is time to make some drinks and take some supplements. Check out these drinks and supplements:

- Supplement: Masulex or Gerovital GH3 – A General and Sexual Rejuvenator
- Supplement: L-Arginine

- Supplement: Melatonin and Pycnogenol

- Green Tea Extract Supplement

Use the Natural Sex Drink listed in the previous chapter.

Here is a juice drink you can prepare to give you protein and a balance of minerals and vitamins.

- 8 oz. of cherry or pomegranate juice
- 2 tablespoons of brewer's yeast
- 2 tablespoons of wheat germ
- 4 tablespoons of desiccated liver

Or, use the drink Paavo Airola, Ph.D., How to Get Well, that is called a sex Pep-up Cocktail, listed above.

Check out the chapter on supplements again and look for other good supplements to use.

Blood Circulation

You will need to make major improvements in your blood circulation or cardiovascular system. It is directly tied to your penis hardness. The more problems you have with your cardiovascular system the more problems you will have with your erections.

All the diets, processes, and nutrients listed here are designed to help you improve your heart and arteries. But you will also need to add to this program exercise.

The pace program is a great program to improve your cardiovascular system without having to spend hours at the gym or exercising at home. So check the exercise chapter again. You may want to check out The Pace Book to get some more ideas on great exercising.

There you have it. You have your work cut out for you. By applying many of the ideas presented here, you will gain a new view of life, and you will get your love life back on track.

Now, you don't have to be doing all of these things at the same time. Start with one of the areas listed above and when you have a good routine doing it, start with another area that you need to do work on.

17: The Author And Other Great Resources

Rudy Silva is a natural nutritional consultant educated in the United States in Nutrition and Physics. He is a graduate of San Jose State University in California. He is the author of 45 other books on natural remedies. He has authored a newsletter in natural remedies for over 10 years.

Resource page

You can see other books about natural remedies that have been written by this author. Go to Google and type in the keyword, Rudy Silva Books.

If you need support or want to promote any of his books, please contact him at rss41@yahoo.com and expect a reply within 24 hours. He looks forward to hearing from you and is happy to help you understand his material on natural and nutritional health.

Give A Review

And, don't forget to give a review for this book so that others can gain the benefits of what is in this book.

To you, for losing weight, creating better health and more happiness in your life,

Rudy S Silva